i

REBUILT RECOVERY

A JOURNEY WITH GOD

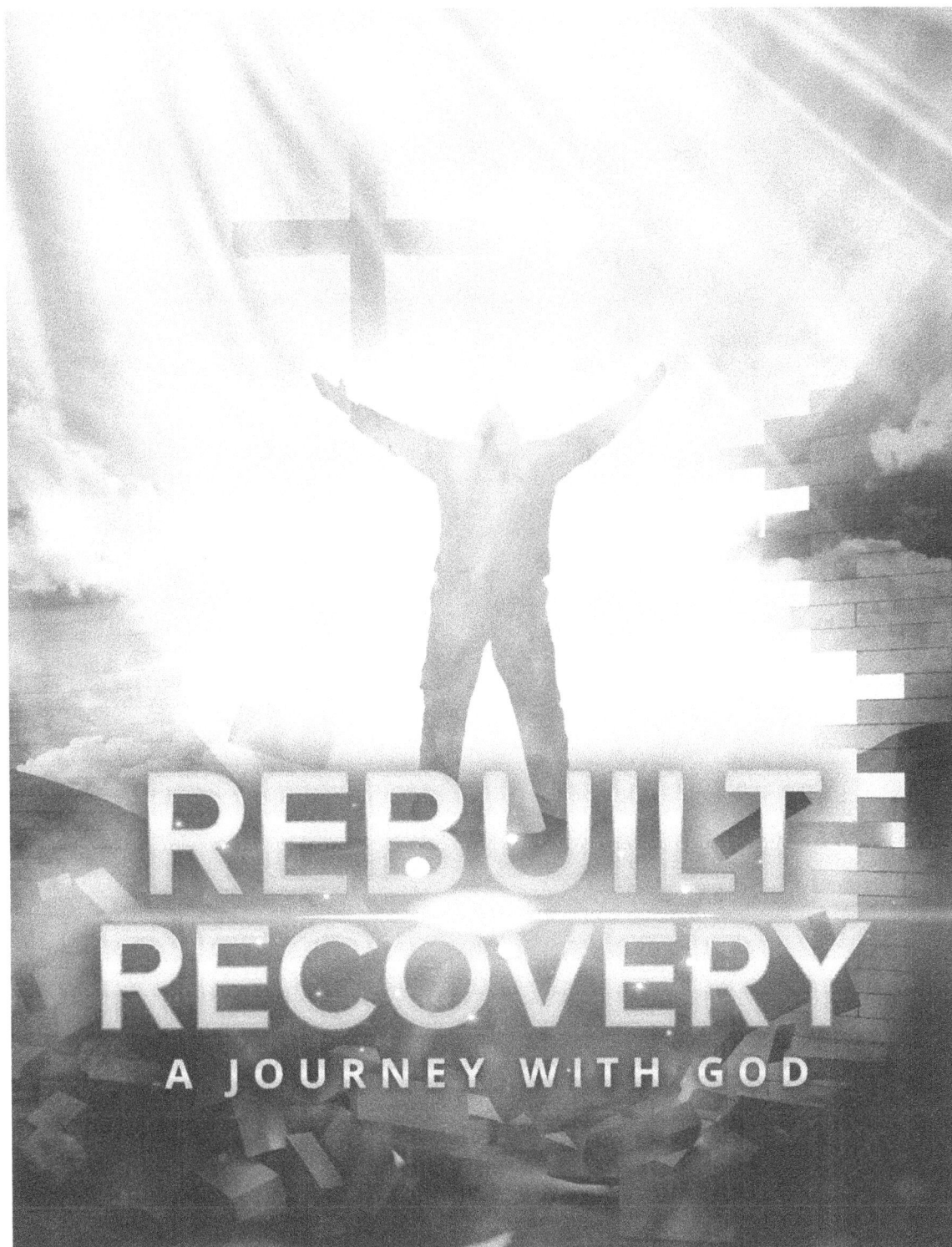

Glorious Hope Publishing

New Carlisle, Ohio

Rebuilt Recovery

A Journey with God

Book 1-4 — Complete Series

By: Heather L. Phipps

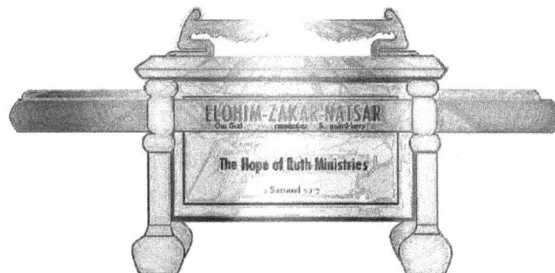

Rebuilt Recovery Is a Ministry of The Hope of Ruth Ministries Church

Glorious Hope Publishing

ISBN: 979-8-9852542-0-4 (Paperback)
ISBN: 979-8-9852542-2-8 (Paperback Black & White)
Library of Congress Control Number: 2021922804

Glorious Hope Publishing
Hope of Ruth Ministries
307 Prentice Dr. New Carlisle, Ohio 45344
info@hopeofruthministries.com
www.hopeofruthministries.com

Thank you to the following people
who gave their ideas, hearts,
and lives into making this book possible.

Cindy Varghese

Summer Curtis

Alysha Allen

Justin Curtis

Annaka Schleinitz-Brooks

Jaycie Curtis

Camie Hawkins

Terri Allison

Contents

Rebuilt Recovery

What Is *Rebuilt Recovery*?

Rebuilt Recovery is a tool to help people find recovery from their mental and emotional pain and suffering by dealing with the root causes of their issues.

Too often, attempts to heal mental health conditions address the symptom of the suffering without looking at the underlying cause. This is especially true with addiction. People often develop addictions in an attempt to mask pain from abuse, neglect, rejection, depression, grief, anxiety, etc. Treating the addiction without first treating the underlying causes feeding the addiction is only a temporary fix. When the person relapses, the problem intensifies, feeding guilt, shame, and feelings of failure that make the original problem even worse.

This is true of other mental disorders as well. OCD, depression, anxiety, schizophrenia, PTSD, or codependency are not the problem. They are the symptom of underlying issues. To treat the mental disorder without treating the cause will end in failure, and an eventual reoccurrence of the symptoms of the disorder.

Rebuilt Recovery is a tool that works in a cooperative effort with the Lord to permanently remove the underlying issues so people may have full healing and receive the joy and freedom promised in Scripture.

What Causes Mental Illness?

Mental illness is complex. The truth is that there is no known, proven cause of mental illness. There is evidence to suggest that your genetic makeup may predispose you to certain mental ailments. This does not mean that you will develop a mental disorder, however; it simply means that it is more likely for you than for someone with a different genetic makeup.

It was once widely thought that the cause of mental disorders was chemical imbalances in the brain. It's true that the chemical balance of the brain does change with depression, anxiety, etc., but this theory, called the chemical imbalance hypothesis, is now widely dismissed by medical professionals. The chemical imbalances in the brain may cause the *symptoms* of these disorders, and medication can aid in easing the symptoms. The cause of the disorder, however, runs much deeper.

What Causes Chemical Imbalances in the Brain?

Chemical imbalances occur when the brain produces natural chemicals called neurotransmitters. The job of the neurotransmitter is to help nerve cells communicate with one another. The way you think creates and reshapes the pathways of this intricate neuro-circuitry in your brain—in other words, your brain physically changes depending on how you are thinking. Your thoughts can literally change the physical structure of your brain. Mental illness is not genetic, but your genetic makeup may put you at a greater risk of developing a mental illness. The way you think about your experiences can activate your genes, so if you are predisposed to mental illness, your thoughts can activate those genetic factors.[1]

---

[1] More information on the science of thinking differently:

https://www.healthline.com/health/chemical-imbalance-in-the-brain

https://www.thebestbrainpossible.com/how-your-thoughts-change-your-brain-cells-and-genes/

https://www.psychologytoday.com/us/blog/bottoms/201611/what-is-cbt

https://www.psychologytoday.com/us/blog/what-mentally-strong-people-dont-do/201710/how-train-your-brain-think-differently

How Do You Heal Mental Disorders?

Physically
Medical professionals may prescribe medicine that works to compensate for the chemical imbalances in your brain as a temporary fix. They may also recommend vitamins, eating well, or exercise, which will improve mood and lead to a better quality of life.

Medicine is a Band-Aid® or a mask; it does not heal you. As your body adapts to medications, the dose must increase to create the same emotional state. Medicines must be used in conjunction with other treatment to be successful.

Mentally
Counselors and therapists use a wide range of therapy techniques such as CBT (Cognitive Behavior Therapy) or CPT (Cognitive Processing Therapy) to change your perspective by training you to consider and reinforce positive beliefs and remove negative beliefs. When successful, there are proven long-lasting results. The solution is to restore the right way of thinking.

Therapies that change the way you think depend on reinforcing your beliefs. The positive thoughts become easier to believe as evidence reinforces the belief. If a belief fails the person, or he lacks evidence for it, destructive thoughts may again lead the person back into emotional instability. A person must base belief on unchangeable truth to effect a permanent change. The Lord is unchanging, and His truth will effect permanent change.

Many methods of treating mental illness often miss the spiritual component. We are not only physical and mental beings; we are also spiritual beings. We have the answer when we know Jesus and the Word.

Spiritually
Churches attempt to address this problem through the concept of faith and works. If you believe enough—have faith—God will heal you. They instruct you in positive behaviors: quit sinning, serve more, live like Jesus, take authority, rebuke the enemy, put on the armor of God. However, churches often neglect the underlying physical and mental components of mental illness, relying only on the spiritual.

Christians have the answer, but many times they fall short in implementation. They often create an expectation of how God will move. People's faith tends to waiver when God does not meet their expectations. They may believe they are not good or spiritual enough for God to heal. Churches only fail if they address one part of the problem without the complete counsel of the Lord. **God's way of healing is found in Scripture and completely addresses mental, physical, and spiritual healing.**

Some Christ-centered recovery groups attempt to combine faith in God's word, living a Christian life, and spiritual warfare with therapy styles to change thought processes. They use Scripture to do this and achieve an excellent success rate. Yet these programs alone do not provide the complete foundational understanding of Scripture and God required to overcome addiction. This may lead people to a faith reliant on the program and not God. Full healing requires recovery and relationship.

Complete Healing
Only with the Lord can you find complete healing. Complete and permanent healing comes when you:
- Discover the root of the problematic thinking
- Replace the negative thinking (the report of the enemy) with truth (the report of the Lord) based on God's unshakable and unchanging truth
- Reinforce the truth with evidence and translate the evidence into belief

Rebuilt Recovery Fills Gaps to Recovery through Scripture!

Complete healing does not mean that you will never experience difficult emotions or temptations. It means you will no longer suffer debilitating emotions or relapse because you have the tools and know-how to work through those difficulties, and you have the joy of the Lord in all circumstances!

Why Is *Rebuilt* Different from Other Recovery Programs?

Christ-centered programs that focus on incorporating a spiritual and mental healing process are successful with those who are solid in their faith. However, these programs tend to neglect to instill a deep, foundational understanding of Scripture, leaving many still searching for the freedom and joy they were promised.

Rebuilt takes recovery to a whole new level. It is personal discipleship mixed with recovery. To be grounded in truth, you must know truth. *Rebuilt Recovery* is a process based on relationship. Why? Because relationship is the basis of everything God is and does. God is relational.

- God is Love (see 1 John 4:8). Love by its very definition requires an object. We are the object of God's love. He created us for the purpose of giving His love to us. Likewise, He desires that we give Him our love.

- God describes our relationship with Himself and other believers using relational language. He is our father, our husband. We are brothers and sisters in Christ, His bride, His child.

- God established people in families to teach us truths about Himself.

The two greatest commandments fulfill all God's laws.

Love the Lord your <u>God</u> with all your heart and with all your soul and with all your strength and with all your mind' and 'Love <u>your neighbor</u> as <u>yourself</u>. (Luke 10:27)

- We are to first love God with our everything.

- We are to love others.

- We are to love ourselves. (This love is not self-centered, but is based on our identity in Christ.)

This is not love as defined by the world. This love It is sacrificial and defined by respect and admiration. This love is the foundational truth on which all Scripture builds. As we build a relationship with God, He teaches us this love, grounding our way of thinking in solid, unshakable truth, which comes from relationship with God. It is that relationship, which transforms our lives, not what we do or believe.

Relationship with God changes our level of faith in Him and provides us evidence of God. It gives us unshakable faith in His ability to provide, protect, guide, heal, and restore. We learn to trust through this relationship. Our faith activates God's power to move in our lives and remove our hurts, provide stability in chaos, and show us hope for the future God prepared for us.

Relationships with others sharpen us, like iron sharpening iron. Healthy relationships provide opportunities to forgive and make amends. God's Word shows us how to choose our relationships wisely, and how to love even people who seem unlovable. God made us for relationship. Nearly all trauma is caused by people, insecurity, or fear of a person's response: rejection, insults, abuse, negligence, crime, loss of people we love, etc. Learning how to relate to people gives us a fresh perspective on what people have done and helps us think about past events differently. Learning to relate to others helps us forgive them and truly release them from their wrong, thus giving us freedom.

Relationship with self allows us to know ourselves as we truly are. We must know ourselves. We must know where we flourish and fail, and we must examine the condition of our hearts. Even more than this, we must love ourselves. This sounds taboo, but Scripture does not say to love other people more than ourselves. God expects humility, but loving others as ourselves implies that we **must** also love ourselves. Because of our sin nature, we do not know how to love ourselves without it becoming a self-seeking kind of love. Scripture shows us how to do this. Loving yourself is seeing yourself through God's eyes, instead of through the lens of your experiences, failures, or your perception of another's opinion of you. It is loving the person God is creating in you as He transforms your heart. Loving yourself overcomes the not _____ enough feelings that come from shame.

What *Rebuilt Recovery* is not

- *Rebuilt Recovery* is not a quick fix. It is a journey with God in a process of healing.

- It is not a 12-step program. It is not a program at all, but a tool.

- It is not responsible for your recovery. God does the healing through your journey.

- It does not take the place of doctors, psychiatrists, or therapists.

- It is not an alternative to medication and does not encourage you to stop medicines or go against any advice a medical care professional has put in place to stabilize you.

- Coaches are not licensed professionals, nor are they responsible for your choices.

- *Rebuilt* is not for people who are not serious about their journey or fully committed to do what God requires for success.

What *Rebuilt Recovery* is

- A tool to guide you on a journey with the Lord through a process of recovery.

- A tool which transforms your lifestyle, drawing you nearer to the Lord and helping you build better relationships so you can relate to God, to others, and to yourself.

- A place of healing and trust, teaching you to develop trust and forgiveness.

- A tool that incorporates biblical principles of recovery, not just behavior modification, using the model of relationship and the "put offs" and "put ons" of Scripture.

Where there is no guidance, a people falls, but in an abundance of counselors there is safety.
(Proverbs 11:14)

The Process

The crucial difference between this journey and other programs is that we approach healing through understanding relationships. The process is relational. This is your path to freedom:

Relationship with God

- Learn that faith is more than simple belief.
- Deal with your doubt and denial.
- Learn to surrender and what that truly means.
- Learn realistic and biblical expectations of God and put to rest false expectations.

Relationships with others

- Understand healthy relationships and their purpose.
- Understand the real meaning of love.
- Learn to have healthy friendships and families.
- Quit avoiding conflict and face your problems, biblically.
- Forgive others for the wrongs they have done against you, so you never have to struggle with them again.
- Learn that forgiveness is something you do once per transgression.
- Make amends for the wrongs you have done to others and experience freedom from your guilt.

Relationship with yourself

- Examine the condition of your heart and learn three biblical "heart checks."
- Learn who you are, where your value and purpose lie, and the character of your God.
- Identify the original source of your emotions and your coping mechanisms.
- Learn to identify and distinguish the truth from the lies you are believing.
- Identify and remove the enemy's strongholds in your life, making the Lord your stronghold.
- Learn the things you must put off before putting on the Armor of God.
- Learn how to love the person God has created you to become.
- Confess the hurts and wrongs in your past and watch them lose their power over you.

The Result

You will know your purpose and have hope for the future again. Your heart will be free from the burdens you have been carrying. You will experience new confidence in yourself and your God. Your faith will become unshakable. Your relationships (as much as it depends on you) will heal. You will handle other people's flaws and their rejection. You will know which people are good for your life and which are not. You will have compassion and love for others, greater than you have ever been able to experience before. You will have an entirely transformed life.

Introduction

Preparing For Your Journey

Welcome to a new season in your life! **This introduction lesson will teach you all you need to begin your journey.** The following lessons are divided into weekly increments to keep you moving and not overwhelmed. Do not be discouraged if you take longer or get stuck. You may require deeper thought or a better frame of mind to move ahead. Some weeks you may be motivated to complete more than one lesson. Go for it! This journey is yours. God and you set the pace, **but it is important to continue despite tough days.**

Rebuilt **is a tool** designed to guide you on a journey of healing with the Lord. Of course, there is no tool, guide, journey, program, recovery, ministry, counselor, preacher, or drug that can fix you. They may help you cope, but only the Lord can fix your brokenness.

Your coach along this journey is your support person, to encourage and strengthen you. You are not walking alone, but your coach cannot make choices for you or heal you. Restoration and healing require a relationship with Jesus Christ and the work of the Holy Spirit.

Listen to the Right Report!

The report of the enemy will try to convince you not to attempt this journey with lies that feed your strongholds of fear, insecurity, and pride. "This will be the same as everything else." "This won't work." "I don't really need this." "I can't trust God to heal me." "I am okay as I am." There is another report, however. **The report of the Lord is truth.** The Lord tells us that He will not forsake us, He will break our chains, freedom is in Him, and by our faith we are healed.

God's responsibility

- ✓ Show you truth about Himself
- ✓ Show you the truth about yourself & your life
- ✓ Love you where you are
- ✓ Heal your heart
- ✓ Forgive your sins
- ✓ Take your life's burdens and place them on His shoulders
- ✓ Remove your fear
- ✓ Give you genuine joy
- ✓ Empower you
- ✓ Strengthen you
- ✓ Give you a purpose
- ✓ Change your heart
- ✓ Make you a new creation

Your responsibility

- ✓ Have faith, believe the Lord will work
- ✓ Be utterly honest with yourself, God, and your coach
- ✓ See it through with complete commitment
- ✓ Choose something different
- ✓ Prepare to change your thoughts about the past, people, & life
- ✓ Be willing to submit everything to the Lord, and make changes

The coach's responsibility

- ✓ Guide you through the questions
- ✓ Share Scripture, personal experiences and insights from their journey with the Lord, etc.
- ✓ Help you see yourself more clearly

What Happens When You Ask the Lord to Join You on Your Journey?

Have you ever heard the story of the prodigal son? It is a type-shadow that shows what happens when one of God's children returns to Him for help. The son did what he wanted, squandering his life and inheritance. He became so desperate that he returned to his father prepared to work as his servant. The father saw him coming and rejoiced, preparing his best to celebrate his son's return. **He accepted the son exactly as he was with open arms of love.**

Starting this journey tells God that you are coming home for help. Oh, how he rejoices! As soon as you begin, He jumps right in with you, walking every step of the way by your side. Regardless of your current relationship with the Lord, He will respond the same way.

Why is this journey necessary? Why does God not just heal everything? God is a gentleman. He will not force your hand or force His way into your life. He allows us to choose Him **and His help**. When we finally humble ourselves enough to ask, He and all the angels in heaven rejoice!

Am I honestly ready to make a commitment to this journey, regardless of what it takes? _____

What may prevent me from making this commitment?

_____

_____

Am I prepared to trust God to do what needs to be done? _____

What makes trusting God difficult for me? _____

*You can begin **even if** you hold on to some doubt. Your honesty, openness and commitment allow your coach to offer suggestions and encouragement.*

Using This Book and Journal

You need a journal. You may use a decorative journal or a simple notebook designated for your *Rebuilt* journey. Some people journal on their computer, although we recommend printing journal pages to keep offline in case something happens to the digital files. Your journal entries will become an invaluable resource. You do NOT want to lose them!

Each lesson has questions for you to answer. Answer the questions as you read. You will discuss the answers when you meet with your coach each week. Use your journal or a separate notebook to record your answers. Write the lesson number and question number before the answer to make it easier to keep your place (i.e., 1.1).

How to Use Your Journal
- Write every day.
- Write your unfiltered thoughts to help sort through clutter in your mind.
- Write about meaningful events during your journey.
- Write about how the Lord is speaking into your life, and His blessings.
- Record your victories! They are vital to remember in hard times.
- Take notes on things to discuss with your coach.
- Write about additional tasks your coach gives along the way.

Your journal is your second most important tool, after the *Rebuilt* books!

Boxes and Symbols

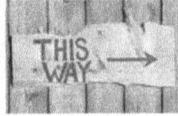

These boxes have thoughts or questions involving your coach.

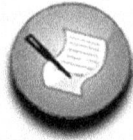

These boxes contain additional tasks for your journey. Do not skip these tasks!

These boxes contain tips with additional information to help understand or implement the topic being discussed.

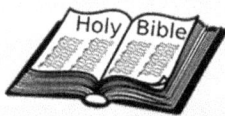

This icon indicates scripture important to understanding the current topic.

These boxes have important points for you to consider.

"These boxes contain interesting quotes"

Disclaimer

The information contained in the *Rebuilt for Life* (online course), *Rebuilt Recovery*, or *Rebuilt Website* is for general information purposes only. The content is not intended to be a substitute for professional advice, diagnosis, or treatment, rather it is intended as a supplement to it. Always seek the advice of your mental health professional or other qualified health provider with any questions you may have regarding your condition. It is your responsibility to inform your mental health professional that you are using a *Rebuilt* service to aid your recovery. Never disregard professional advice or delay in seeking it because of something you have read or heard in *Rebuilt* materials, website, or courses.

> If you are in crisis or have an emergency, call 911 immediately.
>
> **If you have suicidal thoughts, call the National Suicide Prevention Lifeline 1-800-273-TALK (8255) to talk with a skilled, trained counselor at a crisis center in your area.**
>
> **If you are located outside the United States, call your local emergency line immediately.**

***Rebuilt* coaches are not qualified counselors and do not take the place of certified professionals.**

The information is provided by *The Hope of Ruth Ministries* and whilst we endeavor to keep the information up-to-date and correct, we make no representations or warranties of any kind, express or implied, about the completeness, accuracy, reliability, suitability, or availability with respect to the website, books, online course, the information, products, services, or related graphics contained on the internet or print materials for any purpose. Any reliance you place on such information is therefore strictly at your own risk.

In no event will we be liable for any loss or damage including without limitation, indirect or consequential injury, loss, or damage, or any injury, loss, or damage whatsoever arising from loss of life, relations, property, data, or profits arising out of, or in connection with, the use of the *Rebuilt* website, *Rebuilt for Life*, *Rebuilt Recovery*, or *Rebuilt Coaches*.

Every effort is made to keep the websites up and running smoothly. However, *The Hope of Ruth Ministries* nor *Rebuilt Recovery* takes no responsibility for, and will not be liable for, the coaches, website, software, or course being temporarily unavailable due to technical issues beyond our control.

COPYRIGHT NOTICE FOR SUPPLEMENTAL MATERIAL

EXTERNAL LINKS

Through the *Rebuilt* websites and courses, you may link to other websites, which are not under the control of *Rebuilt* or *The Hope of Ruth Ministries*. We have no control over the nature, content, and availability of such sites. The inclusion of any links does not necessarily imply a recommendation or endorse the views expressed within them.

Serenity Prayer

God, grant me the serenity
to accept the things I cannot change,
the courage to change the things I can,
and the wisdom to know the difference.

Living one day at a time,
enjoying one moment at a time;
accepting hardship as a pathway
to peace;

taking, as Jesus did,
this sinful world as it is,
not as I would have it;
trusting that You will make
all things right
if I surrender to Your will;

so that I may be reasonably happy
in this life
and supremely happy with You
forever in the next.

Amen.

Reinhold Niebuhr

Support and Help

You are beginning a new journey with the Lord—most likely, a journey unlike any you have taken before. The Lord can help you all on His own, but that is not His design. God created us to need one another. In His infinite wisdom, God knows when we support others, not only can we guide them, but it also helps us to grow.

As iron sharpens iron, so one man sharpens another.
(Proverbs 27:17)

Your coach will guide you and commit to be there when the road gets bumpy, but additional support is a significant benefit. Accountability partners will keep you on the ideal track and can be available when your coach is not.

The Right People Make All the Difference!

It is important to bring the *right* people along for your journey. Those who accompany you must have your best interests at heart, and trust is essential. The wrong person can lead you astray or encourage you to quit when things get hard. Someone who is judgmental may tear you down and prevent you from being entirely honest with yourself and your coach. Codependents may develop animosity toward your walk as the chains of codependency break.[2]

Family and Friends

Long-standing relationships often have a familiarity that quenches objectivity. It is not always a good option to take close friends or relatives with you on this journey. The people in Jesus' hometown rejected him. To them, he was a mere carpenter's son. They could not accept that Jesus was more than they perceived Him to be.

And Jesus said to them, "A prophet is not without honor, except in his hometown
and among his relatives and in his own household."
(Mark 6:4)

While you are not claiming to be a prophet, you *are* beginning a transformational process in your life. Not everyone will be open to seeing the changes in you.

Choose an Accountability Partner

An accountability partner is an important part of your journey. This is a trusted person who you respect and will be honest with. They must be able and willing to hold you responsible for your journey and keeping on track with your recovery. You must be willing to listen to their counsel, therefore they must be someone who will offer wise, helpful advice and not lead you to temptation. They must be willing to be contacted when you are struggling, even at inconvenient times. It is important to use care when choosing an accountability partner.

---

[2] Codependency is when a person in a relationship controls and manipulates another or depends on the other's needs or control.

Look for the following qualities in an accountability partner:

- Does this person encourage you and lift you up to believe you can be more?

- Does this person have a sincere desire to see you succeed?

- Do you trust this person enough to tell them your innermost secrets? Are they reliable to keep their word?

- Does this person listen well and try to understand you, or do they insist that you agree with their perspective?

- Does this person have a genuine and mature relationship with God?

- Does this person challenge you?

- Does this person have the fortitude and commitment to stand by you in difficult situations?

List some people who might make good accountability partners.

_____

_____

Narrow your options
If you can answer "yes" to any of the following questions about someone you are considering, they should *not* be your accountability partner.

- Does this person gossip or talk about others? If so, they will talk about you also, given the right circumstance.

- Will this person simply agree with you instead of speaking truth you will not want to hear?

- Does the person assume your motives or make comments such as "You always do_____" or "You never_____"? Do they judge your actions because they "know how you are"?

- Will a change in you affect your relationship in a negative or unhealthy way?

- Does this person demean or place guilt on you?

- Does this person create doubt in you and sabotage your success?

- Is this person jealous or threatened by your achievements?

- Is this person argumentative, unable to be wrong, or do they assume they know better than you do?

Write your choice for an accountability partner below.

_____

Ask Someone to Be Your Accountability Partner

Contact the people you chose as potential accountability partners and ask them to come alongside you on your journey. Discuss the following points so they clearly understand what you expect from them.

- You are asking for a commitment to keep you on track and offer support through a challenging year-long journey.

- Sometimes you will need no accountability. Other times you may depend on them daily.

- Your needs may change throughout your journey.

- If you are struggling, you may need them at an inopportune time.

Do not be discouraged if the person you approach refuses, or if you do not know anyone who would make a good accountability partner. If the person you chose does not agree, that is okay. The Lord can bring someone along who is a good fit.

You Are in Charge of Your Journey and Who Gets to Be Part of It!

Sometimes a coach or accountability partner relationship does not work out. This is nothing to worry about. While it is not recommended to leave your coach, if you have trouble relating well with him or her you may ask for someone else. If you are not comfortable with the people supporting you, it will be difficult to succeed.

- Your accountability partner or coach should understand it is not personal if you choose another to walk with you; it is where you are on your journey.

- Do not fear hard feelings when changing a member of your support team.

- Many things can change in a year! Personal situations may prevent someone from being a quality coach or accountability partner. It is better for them to step aside if they cannot be available and consistent.

- You are not required to explain your reasons for requesting a new coach or accountability partner.

- If you fire your coach or if your coach steps away, he or she will help find another to complete your journey with you.

** Coaches are not obligated to fulfill a commitment to people who do not put forth effort, are argumentative, or resist change. These attitudes make a journey ineffective and steal time the coach could spend helping someone ready for the journey. In this situation, a coach will recommend continuing the journey at a later time.

Your Support Team

Copy this page or ask your coach for a copy. Let it remind you to reach out to your support team when you are struggling. Keep it on your refrigerator, desk, or somewhere you will often see it, and keep your coach's information in your phone, wallet, or purse.

If you do not have an accountability partner yet, leave this section blank until you find one.

My *Rebuilt* Coach

Name:
Number:
Email:
Facebook or Other Means of Contact:
Preferred Contact Method:

Accountability Partner

Name:
Number:
Email:
Facebook or Other Means of Contact:
Preferred Contact Method:

Accountability Partner

Name:
Number:
Email:
Facebook or Other Means of Contact:
Preferred Contact Method:

Manage Your Time

Before starting *Rebuilt*, consider how you manage time to prevent becoming overwhelmed by the commitment.

Every purchase has a positive or negative return and a dual cost: the amount spent on the purchase and the hidden cost of everything you cannot get with the money spent. You receive a **positive return** as the property value increases in your home. However, the moment you drive away in a new car, its value depreciates, giving you a **negative return**. A losing lottery ticket is a **total loss**, leaving nothing to show for the money spent. It robbed you of your investment.

> Life's currency is time and energy, and like monetary currency,
> there is a dual cost and return when spent.

Time and energy are your most precious resources. Time is finite and irreplaceable; if we waste it, we cannot regain it. Energy makes time productive. As time passes, less energy is available. When your energy depletes, your time becomes unproductive. You spend more time accomplishing less.

Understanding Wise Investments of Time and Energy

Read the definitions below to familiarize yourself with the terminology:

- **A Return** refers to positive or negative impact from investing time or energy.

- **A Positive Return** is when our effort adds an element of quality, surplus of energy, or redeems the investment for our benefit.

- **A Negative Return** brings harm to us or others, leaving us worse off for our effort.

- **Robbed of Time/Energy** implies an investment that steals time or is a complete loss. This includes mind-numbing activities like social media or television, non-productive time spent daydreaming or worrying, and investing time in someone who does not reciprocate or benefit from your investment.

We spend time and energy in four areas. To learn more about these four areas, read the descriptions below and answer the questions.

1. **Physical Investment** — Our activities are an obvious investment of time and energy. Exercising, walking, cleaning, cooking, working, traveling, sleeping, eating, or being sick, all cost time and energy. Physical investments such as laughing, crying, and fits of rage may also have an emotional investment such as joy, grief, and anger. This is a dual investment. Many times, our physical investments **return a positive benefit**. We exercise and our bodies become stronger. We go to work and earn money. When we help another, we receive joy. Sometimes, our physical investments give us a **negative return**. We fall behind when we waste time doing the wrong things. We lose opportunities when we are not wise in how we spend our time. Negative actions, such as yielding to addiction or gluttony of food or pleasure, provide a negative return to our health, our mental and emotional state, and even our wallets.

1) Consider what you do. What are your greatest physical investments?

2) What is the time and energy cost of your physical investments?

3) Describe the negative returns on your physical investments.

4) What positive returns result from your physical investments?

5) In what ways do your physical investments rob you of time and energy?

2. **Emotional Investment** — Emotions influence our investment of time and energy into people, dreams, goals, grudges, and ourselves. We may spend a great deal of time and energy fighting, denying, or avoiding emotions. Emotional investments may bring joy and a sense of worth, or leave us drained with rage, grief, and sadness, as hidden violations and unforgiveness fester in our hearts.

Questions to Ponder

6) What are your emotional investments?

7) How do your emotional investments spend time and energy?

8) In a typical week, how often are your feelings negative? How often are they positive?

9) Do your emotional time and energy investments have a positive or negative return?

10) How do your emotions steal your time and energy?

3. **Mental Investment** — Many things require a mental investment of our time and energy: thinking, worrying, planning, researching, studying, writing, daydreaming, reading books, watching videos, or playing games. Dwelling on negative or ignoble things can drain our energy and rob us of our time or give us a negative return on our time. However, meditating on things of the Lord—His blessings, purpose, and future—can give us the positive returns of hope, encouragement, and motivation. When we rest our mind in the Lord, He renews our strength and energy.

Questions to Ponder

11) What are your mental investments?

12) How do your mental investments spend your time and energy?

13) Is your thinking mostly positive (hopeful), negative (pessimistic), or neutral?

14) What thoughts give you a positive or negative return?

15) What thoughts give you no return, robbing you of your time and energy?

4. **Spiritual Investment** — A spiritual life requires time and energy. We seek spiritual wellbeing to find meaning, purpose, and security in life. Investing time and energy in a relationship with God fills our spiritual needs. The Lord renews our energy, gives us rest, and redeems our time. When we seek to fill our spiritual needs from different sources—such as nature, self, money, or idols—our investment returns void or empty of meaning. Our drive to seek purpose and meaning exhausts our energy.

<u>Questions to Ponder</u>

16) How much time and energy do you spend in prayer, devotion, church, witnessing to others, worship, Bible reading, or meditating and listening to the Lord?

17) What other spiritual influences are in your life? (E.g., horoscopes, fantasy, spiritualism apart from the Lord, books, movies, etc.)

18) What is the return on your spiritual investments? What percentage of your return is negative, positive, or both?

19) Are there any negative influences you allow to take up your spiritual time and energy? Are you aware of the impact and cost to you?

20) How do spiritual investments steal your time and energy?

Now, consider this next set of questions to help you break down the cost of your time and energy and how that cost affects your life.

<u>Questions to Ponder</u>

21) **Estimate the percentage of your time spent in each category.** (For example: 40% Physical, 25% Emotional, 30% Mental, 5% Spiritual.)

22) **Estimate the percentage of your energy spent in each category.**

23) **What investments give a positive return?**

24) **What are the benefits of the positive returns you identified?**

25) **What investments give a negative return?**

26) **What harm comes from the negative returns you identified?**

27) **Which investments leave you robbed, unable to identify a return or loss?**

28) **What losses have you identified resulting from the way you invest your time and energy?**

29) **How are you spending more time and energy than you have available to give?**

30) **How could you invest less time and energy in the things that rob you or give a negative return?**

31) **How could you invest more time and energy in the things with a positive return?**

32) **Is there any investment that causes a negative return or loss, which you can invest differently to create a positive return?**

Let's Begin

God is ready to embark on this journey with you. Give Him your trust one day at a time and watch as He increases your faith. When experiencing hard times, do not fear failing or that you lack the faith to succeed. Remember your commitment and move forward anyway. It is in these times that the Lord proves Himself faithful. This journey will cover steep hills and deep valleys, but you never walk alone. For every difficult moment, there is an equally exciting victory!

Say a Prayer

Would you embark on a trip with friends without first discussing it? Of course not! This is no different. Take a moment to pray, asking the Lord to accompany you on your journey. In reality, you are not inviting Him to come with you, but requesting to go with Him. He is the one leading your journey.

Are you unsure how to pray? *Rebuilt* does not script prayers, as they must be a genuine reflection of your heart. If you struggle to find the words, consider the suggestions below to guide your prayer:

- Thank the Lord for your blessings and this opportunity.
- Repent and seek forgiveness if something weighs on your mind.
- Commit to seeking healing in His ways.
- Ask the Lord to reveal Himself through this journey.
- Ask the Lord to search your heart to uncover any denial.
- Share any doubt, lack of faith, or unbelief with the Lord.
- Pray regarding any concerns you have about beginning this journey.
- Ask the Lord keep you accountable, honest, and committed.

Ready,
Set,
Begin!

Introduction to Book One

Prepare the Way

As with any journey, you must prepare before you leave: Plan the route, pack the right supplies, and choose your travel companions. It is the same way on a spiritual journey!

Plan Your Path
Your path is set before you. Consider this guide your GPS.

Pack for the Journey
You will travel light. All you need is a Bible, this guide, a journal (or two or three ...), and pens or pencils.

Your Travel Companions
You will travel with the Lord, whose spirit will minister to you and teach you throughout your journey, and with your coach, who will be there to keep you focused on the Lord and give some encouragement along the way. Once you get started, you may make a pit stop and ask one or two trusted friends to come along on the journey. They can give additional support and help keep you accountable.

Plan Adventures and Sight-seeing
There will be many destinations along the way, and it will be the greatest adventure of your life. You will see many sights as your eyes become opened to the truth. But as with everything, there are guidelines to follow:

- Be completely honest with yourself, your coach, and God. The road becomes bumpy and treacherous when you break this rule.
- Never give up. Quit the journey early, and you may end up stranded in the wilderness without a ride home.
- Do not isolate yourself. You can easily get lost in unfamiliar territory if you pull away from your coach or from God. You do not want to be stuck in the wilderness!

Method of Transportation
One step at a time. You can walk through the books at your own pace, just do not stop moving. Your coach will go over your answers to the questions in the book, your journal (if you want to share), and answer questions along the way.

- Meetings with your coach are confidential, so you can be free to share whatever is on your mind. (Your coach will discuss this in more detail with you).
- Pray before working through the books and listen for the Lord.
- Each day, journal about your feelings, concerns, or what the Lord is teaching you.

Chapter One

Faith

Lesson 1 — Defining Faith

Questions to Ponder

1.1) To begin a journey with the Lord requires faith. Before we look at what the scriptures say, take a minute and write in your notebook or journal what you believe faith is, and what it requires of you.

1.2) Is a belief that Jesus existed, died, and rose again the only thing required for salvation?   If your answer is no, then explain what else is required.

1.3) In your understanding, what does it mean to know Jesus?

What Does Scripture Say?

Scripture uses the words *faith* and *belief* similarly, but when we consider belief, we often see it from a narrow perspective. Let us look at the most famous passage in all of Scripture, John 3:16:

> *For God so loved the world, that he gave his only Son, that whoever believes in him should not perish but have eternal life.*

This verse by itself seems to say that all salvation requires is to believe that Jesus existed, and that He died and rose from the grave. Some view anything else as works and not a requirement for salvation. However, no single verse of Scripture was ever intended to be the only word of God on a matter. We must consider the whole counsel of God. The Lord expresses that there is more to relationship with Him than the simple belief Jesus exists when he says this:

> *Many will say to Me on that day, "Lord, Lord, did we not prophesy in Your name, and in Your name cast out demons, and in Your name perform many miracles?" And then I will declare to them, "I never knew you; depart from me you who practice lawlessness." (Matthew 7:21 – 23)*

The Lord describes people who believed in Him, even used His name to perform miracles—yet Jesus says to them, "I do not know you." Realizing that the name of Jesus has power and knowing Scripture are not sufficient to save us. We must **know Him**.

What Does It Mean to Believe? What Is Faith?

Hebrews 11 tells us what God means when He speaks of faith in Scripture. Faith is confidence or **trust** in what our senses cannot perceive. It is assurance of our hopes.

> *Now faith is confidence in what we hope for and assurance about what we do not see. (Hebrews 11:1)*

We all have had experiences where we realize God has come through for us, and times we feel He disappointed us. Many times, our disappointment comes because we cannot see the whole picture. We cannot understand why our prayers were not answered the way we assumed they should be answered. This can cause us to doubt God.

Do not worry if you struggle to answer the lesson questions. Mistakes are where learning happens! Sometimes we cannot know the answers, or the answers come later. The important thing is to understand that just because we do not have all the answers, we **can** still have full confidence in our God.

What Faith Looks Like

We know that **without faith it is impossible to please God** (Hebrews 11:6). The rest of Hebrews 11 shows examples of the attitudes and actions of faith. Unwavering trust allows us to be obedient to God even when, in our own wisdom, we cannot make sense of His commands.

Read Hebrews 11

Questions to Ponder

1.4) When, if ever, did you put your trust or hope in God for a situation that you could not control or understand?

    a. Was the outcome what you thought you wanted? Was the outcome better or worse than you expected? How did this situation change your level of trust in God?

    b . Did the outcome of the situation disappoint your expectations? How did this change your level of trust in God?

1.5) Are you willing to look at situations in which God did not answer your prayers the way you wanted from a new perspective? Can you see any other possible reasons for the way the Lord responded to your prayers?

Examples of Living a Life of Faith

The people mentioned in Hebrews 11 are examples of living a life of faith. They **lived by faith** until they died. Even if they **did not see the result** of the promise, they set their minds on eternity and were Kingdom-minded. **God was unashamed** of them and counted them as righteous because of their faith. Their faith was not a simple belief, but a faith that produced obedience.

Each person in Hebrews 11 had sin and major life mess-ups, yet God calls them all righteous.

- Noah became so drunk one night that his son Ham caught him passed out and naked.

- Abraham, the "father of our faith," falsely claimed that his wife was his sister to escape harm.

- Moses murdered an Egyptian, feared speaking to pharaoh, and had a temper problem.

From Hebrews 11 we learn that faith is

- A belief that Jesus exists

- An earnest seeking after Him

- Demonstrated through sincere offerings

- The fear of the Lord
- A knowing that God is a God of His word, trusted and respected
- Obedience, even when we do not understand the why
- To go where God sends us
- To believe God is faithful to us, that his word is true **for us**
- To know God's promises **will be fulfilled**, even if we do not see the result in our lifetime
- To stay hopeful because we set our minds on the things of the Kingdom, of eternity, not things of this world
- To suffer and persevere with Christ
- Not fearing the world's ridicule, imprisonment, even death, because our faith is in that which is eternal

Faith is relational!

Questions to Ponder

1.6) Do you ever think your sin may keep God from helping you? Is this truth?

1.7) Looking at the list from Hebrews 11, in which areas is your faith strong?

1.8) Are there areas where you cannot trust God?

Faith Activates God's Power

Our faith, as defined by the Word of God, moves the Lord to activate His power in our lives. The Lord guarantees that when we trust and submit our journey to Him, He **will** change our lives and heal us from hurts and strongholds keeping us stuck. Sometimes it is hard to trust, and this allows doubt to creep in.

> *But let him ask in faith, with no doubting, for the one who doubts is like a wave of the sea that is driven and tossed by the wind. For that person must not suppose that he will receive anything from the Lord; he is a double-minded man, unstable in all his ways. (James 1:6 – 8)*

Trust Is an Act of Love

Trust is a gift, which is an act of love. When we give God our trust, we are showing him love. It is an act of love because trust is sacrificial. To give even that small amount of faith makes us vulnerable, because the one to whom we are giving faith may fail us. We may get hurt. Faith is a selfless act of love and trust, and the greatest gift we can give God. We do nothing in our own power; the only thing we have control over is our choices. We cannot even choose God without Him drawing us in.

> *No one can come to me unless the Father who sent me draws him. And I will raise him up on the last day. (John 6:44)*

The choice we really need to make is whether we will trust the Lord. Even a small amount of trust will do a lot. When we learn about Christ and dig into His word, we make a choice to believe.

So faith comes from hearing, and hearing through the word of Christ. (Romans 10:17)

Questions to Ponder

1.9) How do you struggle with doubt?

1.10) What are your Bible study habits? Do you trust the Word of God?

1.11) List any questions about God or the Bible that are a stumbling block to your faith.

1.12) Are you willing to give the Lord an opportunity to prove He is trustworthy? What would that look like for you?

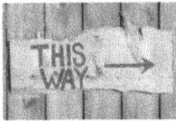

Work with your coach on your tough questions! Do not be afraid to ask your coach anything. If they do not know the answer, they will help you find it! Did you do the Time Management exercise in the Getting Started section? Review it with your coach!

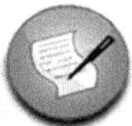

- Make it a habit to start each lesson in this workbook in prayer. Pray each morning about this journey you are taking.
- Ask to walk with the Lord throughout your day.
- Ask the Lord to guide you as you answer the questions in your notebook.
- Pray each evening about your day. Listen for the Lord to give you understanding. Write about it in your journal.

Chapter Two

Deal with Your Doubt

Lesson 2 — Dealing with Doubt

No person increases our faith—not a pastor, mentor, or even ourselves. It is the Lord who gives the increase when we reach out with the smallest seed of faith.

> *So neither he who plants nor he who waters is anything, but only God who gives the growth. … You are God's field, God's building. (1 Corinthians 3:7,9)*

The apostles realized this and asked the Lord to increase their faith.

> *The apostles said to the Lord, "Increase our faith!" And the Lord said, "If you had faith like a grain of mustard seed, you could say to this mulberry tree, 'Be uprooted and planted in the sea,' and it would obey you." (Luke 17:5 – 6)*

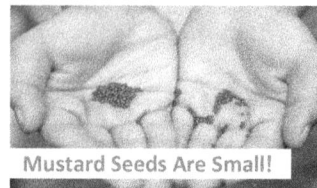

Mustard Seeds Are Small!

Jesus tells them that if they had even a little amount of faith (a mustard seed is very tiny), they could do the impossible. In other passages, Jesus scolds his disciples for not having enough faith. Yet in each case, He is telling them to simply believe. You can know something is true in your head, but believing it with all your heart is far more difficult.

We already know that faith comes by hearing the Word, so studying Scripture is a great place to start. **After all, how do you trust in a God you do not know?**

How does faith grow?
- By reading the Word
- Through testing and trial
- With prayer

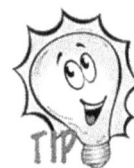

Opportunity to Use Our Faith

God will give us opportunities to use our faith, testing our faith in trials. When everything is going well, it is easy to have faith in God, but the true demonstration of our faith is when the trials come. Do we trust God, put it in his hands, and believe for a victorious outcome, or do we try to control matters ourselves and thus fall into worry, panic, or fear?

> *In this you rejoice, though now for a little while, if necessary, you have been grieved by various trials, so that the tested genuineness of your faith—more precious than gold that perishes though it is tested by fire—may be found to result in praise and glory and honor at the revelation of Jesus Christ. (1 Peter 1:6 – 7)*

> *Count it all joy, my brothers, when you meet trials of various kinds, for you know that the testing of your faith produces steadfastness. And let steadfastness have its full effect, that you may be perfect and complete, lacking in nothing. (James 1:2 – 4)*

Of course, we can pray for the Lord to help us. Do you remember how the apostles asked the Lord to increase their faith? There are many stories of people of God who struggled at times to trust God. When we ask God to help us with our doubt, it gives him permission to work in our lives, increasing our faith.

Consider the story of the boy possessed by a demonic spirit from his early childhood (see Mark 9:14 – 29). The father was weak in faith, but he asked Jesus to help his son. The father said, "But *if* you can do anything, have compassion on us and help us." And Jesus said to him, "***If you can***! All things are possible for one who believes." Immediately the father of the child cried out and said, "***I believe; help my unbelief!***"

This man cried out to Jesus in doubt, but Jesus responded to him that it would be possible if he would believe. The father realized his doubt. He told Jesus he believed and asked for help with his unbelief. Jesus made it a point to show this man that it is **not** about what **Jesus** could do. (After all, Jesus was given all authority in heaven and earth. See Matthew 28:18). It was about what the man could do. **Could he believe?** The man wanted the kind of faith that pleased Jesus and asked Him to help with his unbelief. Jesus honored his effort to trust, meeting him where he was, and He healed the boy. He will do the same for us. He meets us in our unbelief.

Never hesitate to pray for help when you struggle with doubt and unbelief!

Denial

Denial is not the same as doubt. In denial, you refuse to look at part of yourself or your life honestly. This is a detrimental coping skill. Denial can show itself many ways:

- By minimizing a difficult time of life as being in the past and over, without ever addressing how it made us feel or the way it impacted how we respond to situations today.

- By ignoring a character flaw ("I'm not so bad; at least I'm not like_____!")

- By hiding a sin or issue in our family because of shame and embarrassment

- By drawing attention to another's flaws to draw attention away from our own issues

- By projecting negativity

- By burying how we feel in medication, illegal drugs, or alcohol

Questions to Ponder

2.1) **Make a plan to help grow your faith. Include studying the Word, how you will pray, and what you will do during a trial. Put your plan into action this week.**

2.2) **How are you going about daily praying and journaling? If you struggle to do this every day, write how you are struggling and a plan to help you be more consistent.**

Forget the Past

We should **not** hang onto the past, but the only way to truly overcome it is to deal with it. Then we can move ahead, leaving the pain of the past behind us. Paul says in Philippians 3:13,

Brothers, I do not consider that I have made it my own. But one thing I do: forgetting what lies behind and straining forward to what lies ahead.

Some people use this verse as a reason not to dig up the past, thinking that doing so is merely being a victim, continually obsessed with what has happened to them. However, Paul is telling us to keep our eyes on where we are going, instead of looking back to where we have been. **He is not telling us to ignore the past**.

> When you are in denial, refusing to look at or deal with the things that hurt you in the past, there are lasting consequences.
>
> The result is that you cannot move forward, and **you are in fact living in the oppression of your past,** regardless of whether you can admit it or not.
>
> Refusing to deal with past situations leaves you trapped there.

Hanging onto our past is not always something we do knowingly!

Consequences of Denial

When you deny or discount your feelings, all your emotions become muted. Suppressed emotions can cause anxiety, expressing themselves as unexplainable fear and fatigue. Not only do we mute the bad feelings; we also silence the good ones. This can lead to depression. There is freedom in experiencing our emotions, even when the feelings are unpleasant.

Denial is as if you are running away from your past
yet terrified of stepping into your future.

Questions to Ponder

2.3) Can you identify coping skills that you use now (or have used in the past) to deal with shame, fear, pain, insecurity, depression, etc.? How do you handle difficult situations?

2.4) What have you clung to for way too long? Anger? Fear? Loneliness? Unforgiveness? Resentments? Or something else?

Many people do not realize they have unmet expectations. Denial of your expectations may cause tension in your relationships and make you feel impatient and irritated. Even when you get what you thought you wanted, you still may not feel satisfied or find yourself complaining that nothing works out. Your denial causes you to live in the lie that you can somehow achieve the unreasonable expectations you place on yourself.

Denial is the lie that keeps us trapped **indefinitely**. It tells us we are safe from our past with our "yuck" buried behind vast walls no one can penetrate. But the people who have "walked in your shoes" can see right through those walls.

In denial, we think we are hidden, but we are simply blind.

Have you ever heard the saying, "You are only as sick as your secrets"? Your secrets are anything you deny and keep hidden in the dark. Bring those secrets into the light, and they lose their power over you. God promises us that while we are blind and stuck, He will guide us out of our darkness.

And I will lead the blind in a way that they do not know, in paths that they have not known I will guide them. I will turn the darkness before them into light, the rough places into level ground. These are the things I do, and I do not forsake them.
(Isaiah 42:16)

Questions to Ponder

2.5) Fear can take many forms: Jealousy, insecurity, anxiety, worry, control, etc. In what ways do you experience fear?

2.6) Consider recent situations where you were wronged or felt uncomfortable. What was your emotional response? (Did you feel insecure, angry, fearful, panicked, sad/depressed, lonely/empty, numb, etc.?)

2.7) Take an honest look at yourself. Can you identify the walls you present to others?

2.8) What are your secrets? (These can include family secrets.) Bring them into the light!

Today, commit to breaking out of your walls of denial.

Pray and speak to the Lord about your choice.
Ask him to search your heart and show you anything you missed.

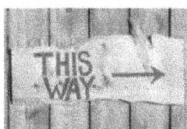

Do you struggle to pray and journal?
Ask your coach to help you come up with a
plan to be consistent!

Chapter Three

Surrender

Lesson 3 — Why Surrender?

Surrender

Most likely, if you are on this journey, you have been trying to get your life under control and finally decided to do something different. You will get a grip on your life once and for all!

What if, to gain a grip on your life, you had to loosen your grip on it?
Does that sound counter-productive—even crazy—to you?

The two principal reasons we refuse to surrender are pride and control. Pride separates us from God, and He expects us to give Him control.

Surrender is letting go, but what does that really mean? How does that work? Before you can let something go, you must identify what you are holding on to. Start examining how you handle life now. **Take your time** to answer these questions about your life and **answer as honestly** as you can.

We have discussed how faith is crucial for our relationship with God and our journey. Surrender is also crucial. **God is a gentleman.** He takes nothing you are not willing to give.

Questions to Ponder

3.1) In what areas of your life are you holding onto regret? (Had I only made a different choice, everything would be different …)

3.2) What things have you been doing again and again in an effort to improve your life?

3.3) When have you made poor choices because your emotions led you, and what was the result?

3.4) What kinds of things have you done to ease or lessen pain in your heart?

3.5) List the things about which you are currently (or most) angry and resentful. How are these things affecting your life?

3.6) Where are you getting your purpose and value?

3.7) List all the positive labels that describe you. (Smart, beautiful, artist, designer, etc.)

3.8) List all the negative labels that describe you. (Stupid, fat, lazy, unpopular, rejected, selfish, ugly, etc.)

3.9) In what ways are you selfish or prone to putting yourself before others?

Control

Control prevents surrender. Why do we refuse God access to part of our life, and fight Him for control? We covet control because we want things our way. We do not trust that God's way is best or that it will please us. We may fear His desires will not match our own, or that He may ask of us something we are not willing to give. Yet when we give over control, life becomes easier as we lose the burden of that responsibility. Complete surrender means we no longer need to worry because God will provide our needs. If we walk and abide with Him, we **will** do right by Him.

I am the vine; you are the branches. Whoever abides in me and I in him, he it is that bears much fruit, for apart from me you can do nothing. (John 15:5)

Powerless

In your flesh, you are powerless to do what is right and will always fall into sin. In your own wisdom, you will mess up every time. Your flesh pursues pleasure, often in sin, but happiness from worldly pursuits is always temporary. It lasts only a moment before you need to find something even bigger and greater to make you happy, and that too is short-lived. **The flesh can never be satisfied.** It will always want more and leave us searching our entire lives for fleeting moments of rest and happiness.

Strength and Wisdom

The Lord gives us joy, which is better than happiness. Bad things happen to both "good" and "bad" people. With the Lord's joy in our lives, we can ride out life's storms in peace. Joy does not end, but happiness does. **You can have joy in difficult moments, even when you cannot have happiness.** The joy of the Lord gives us the strength, the ability to persevere and the desire to be and do more.

Wisdom is another source of strength in the Lord. In our own wisdom we only understand in part, from our limited perspective. We misunderstand people, become offended, fall into traps, and fail. However, the Lord knows everyone's heart. He sees the past, present, and future. He knows the beginning and the end of every situation you find yourself in, and the Lord always speaks truth. To live in His wisdom is to be strong in your life.

Why would you ever want to use your own wisdom?
Why would you not want to give over control?

! God Has Expectations

There are several things God expects from us. The most important are to **have faith** (trust), and **to surrender** to His will (give Him control). The more faith we have, the easier it is to give up our control. We must relinquish our shortcomings (sin and strongholds), so we can see clearly to help other believers do the same. It is through God that we overcome strongholds.

You hypocrite, first take the log out of your own eye, and then you will see clearly to take the speck out of your brother's eye. (Matthew 7:5)

He expects our trust and obedience, that we will judge others fairly, and offer people forgiveness when they hurt us. These four things develop in us **a heart like Christ, full of love**, and love is the point of everything. Without love we are nothing. *(1 Corinthians 13:3).*

3.10) What do you have control over in your life?

3.11) In what areas do you lack control?

3.12) Are there areas of your life that you fear giving God control over? List them. For each item, describe what you are afraid of.

Do we have control?

There is exceptionally little that we control. Most circumstances in life come about because of other people's choices, the government, or natural disasters (storms, fire, etc.), or any number of other causes. Out of everything we think we can control, we will find we can only control two things:

We have control over our thoughts and our choices. That is all!

In the previous questions, you may have mentioned situations where you are "in charge," such as if you manage employees at your work. The fact is that you may oversee your employees or children, but do you really have control over them? You can make choices to discipline them, to coerce compliance, but the choice to listen to your authority is theirs. You cannot control their choices. There really is not much we can control on this earth. We can possibly influence things and people, but we cannot control them.

Question to Ponder

3.13) What areas of your life are you willing to release your grip on and hand over to the Lord?

3.14) Review the "Stop, Drop, and Roll" strategy on the next page, and use it this week. Then write about how well it worked for you or about any difficulties using the strategy.

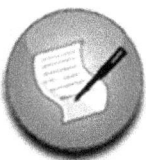

- **Do not forget to write about your day each evening in your journal.**
- **Write about areas of your life that have been holding you down.**
- **Write about unreasonable expectations or control issues you may have.**
- **Spend some quiet time studying the Word.**
- **Ask the Lord what He wants you to Surrender to Him.**

Strategy: Stop, Drop, and Roll

Every bad choice begins with a wrong thought. It may seem difficult to believe that you have control over your thoughts, but you do—and stopping wrong thinking is vital to your recovery! You may not be able to stop a thought from entering your mind, but you can control how that thought affects you. The Word says to take your thoughts captive and make them obedient to the Lord. This implies that you should be aware of your thoughts. Dismiss wrong thinking and replace those thoughts with God's truth.

This strategy can help you prevent a crisis in any situation before it starts. Remember your fire safety lessons from school? They taught you if you are on fire, you must stop where you are, drop to the ground, and roll to smother the fire. Instead of a physical fire, we are going to teach you to put out symbolic fires in your thinking that can cause devastating burns.

Stop

Stop and think. No matter what situation comes up, stop and think before you act. Stay aware of your thoughts throughout the day. Pay attention to emotional responses and see if you can identify the thought behind the response. What are you thinking? Is your self-talk detrimental? Are you leaning on the Lord in the situation, or on your own strength?

Drop

Drop the lie. If you find your thinking goes against what you are learning from the Lord, you are on "fire." Identify the lie. Would the Lord say the same thing to you that you are saying to yourself? Would you give another person the advice you are speaking to yourself? Are your thoughts degrading you or another person? Test the thought with Scripture!

Roll

Roll with the truth. Find the truth in the situation. Are you misunderstanding something? Pray for understanding and the Lord's wisdom on what to do. If you are distraught, seek the peace of the Lord through worship. Sometimes the lies in our mind shout so loudly they drown out the truth. If you must, shout the truth aloud until it is louder than the lies in your mind. You may get some strange looks, but it works!

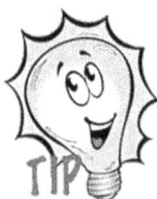

If you are unsure of God's truth for a particular situation, you can use tools such as

https://www.openbible.info/

to search Scripture for any topic you can imagine. Pray and ask the Holy Spirit to reveal the truth to you.

Lesson 4 — Identifying Expectations

Expectations

Expectations are some of the most **difficult things to surrender.** Everyone has expectations. We have expected things of people and carried the burden of other's expectations since we were young children. Sometimes we expect too much of ourselves, and other times we wear ourselves down trying to meet another person's unreasonable expectations. We may experience guilt when failing to live up to standards another sets, and sometimes we believe even God expects more than we can give. Examining expectations will help you discover areas you need to surrender.

Sometimes people want so much from us that it becomes a stress on our daily lives. We must learn to identify unfair expectations but **realize that not all expectations are harmful.** They may keep us motivated and accountable and help us set goals or make plans.

> ### Question to Ponder
> **4.1) Who places expectations on you? What are those expectations? (Be sure to include family, church, pastors, employers, friends, coworkers, and everyone you interact with regularly.)**

Expectations of self

When our expectations of ourselves are too high to meet, we may feel like a failure or that we cannot be good enough. Are you expecting perfection of yourself? Do you expect to accomplish more than your time allows? Are any of your expectations unnecessary? If you expect more of yourself than you can give, **especially** if others do **not** hold you to the same standard, you must evaluate your expectations.

Sometimes **we do not expect enough** from ourselves. This does not necessarily imply laziness, but it may indicate that you feel that you are not smart enough, talented enough, brave enough, or good enough to meet a higher expectation. Are there areas of your life where you should expect more of yourself?

> Evaluate this carefully. Would you hold others to the same expectations you set for yourself, or do you expect more from others than you are willing to give?

Do you expect people to be your security, approval, value, purpose, confidence, love, or trust? Do others expect this of you? If you expect another to fill these holes in your life, you may blame them for your lack. In truth, you cannot count on another person to fill these gaps. People are flawed, and they are not designed to meet these needs. Eventually, they will fail you. If another expects this from you, you will fail them. These needs are holes in our life that can only be filled by God—the only one who will never fail.

Analyze Your Expectations

Think about the expectations you identified in question 4.1. Try to see the reason behind these expectations from the other person's perspective. Is the expectation a responsibility to your family or a boss? Does the expectation have a positive impact or benefit on your life? **These are most likely reasonable expectations**.

On the other hand, do other people's expectations arise from selfish motives or take advantage of you? Are they more than you can give? Are the expectations placed on you different from the expectations placed on another in your position? Is it something another person would consider unfair or unreasonable if you asked them to do the same thing? If you said "yes" to any of these questions, **then they are probably unreasonable expectations**.

Questions to Ponder

4.2) Think about the expectations you identified in question 4.1 from the other person's perspective. Are any of these expectations unreasonable?

4.3) Are these expectations hurting you (physically, emotionally, spiritually)? Describe How.

4.4) How should you handle these unreasonable expectations?

4.5) Now consider the expectations you put on yourself. Write a complete list of these expectations. Who else expects you to achieve these expectations?

4.6) What personal expectations should you reevaluate?

4.7) In what areas of your life can and should you expect more from yourself?

4.8) In what areas of your life do you lack confidence? How could you strengthen confidence in yourself?

4.9) Do you blame any of your problems on things that are missing from your life? What are those things?

4.10) What or who have you used to fill those gaps in your life?

Lesson 5 — Down with Pride

There are many other reasons we refused to hand control over to God. Here are some that might sound familiar:

- We want things our own way. We want what we want, and we do not want God to do something different.

- We enjoy our sin and do not want to change it.

- We worry about what others will think about us or what we are doing.

- We are afraid. A common first response to fear is to want to take control.

- We assume we know what is best.

These ways of thinking are birthed by fear and pride. Fear is a lie of the enemy. We fear not having what we want or losing opportunities. Sometimes we fear we will miss out on something fun. We fear people's opinions because we are afraid to offend and fear rejection. We think we know better, and that listening to God or another's advice will not produce our desired result. We need not be afraid. God can take better care of us and our loved ones than we ever could.

Pride

Pride is not just thinking more of yourself than you should. It manifests in many ways. Most of us understand pride as when we think we have better, do better, or are better than another person. Pride is also when we think we are better, know better, or can do better than God. We display our pride many ways:

- Not following rules or laws

- Refusing to listen or hear sound counsel

- Being judgmental and comparing ourselves to others

- Seeking to control a situation

- Bossiness, or demanding that others think and act our way

- Conceit, arrogance, and self-praise

- Selfishness

- Vengefulness

- Teasing and mockery

- Gossip and seeking "dirt" on someone, or harboring evil suspicions

- Rejecting those in different economic, racial, political, or other groups

- Causing disputes about words to prove we are correct

- Stirring up controversial arguments, etc.

Have you ever met someone who often degrades themselves, cannot be comforted, speaks and acts like a victim, or constantly complains about how they are treated? These people, living in a state of continuous humiliation, may in fact be prideful, desiring praise and attention. Their false humility can be a form of manipulation to get others to feed their pride.

Pride prevents surrender and separates us from God. There are hundreds of scriptures dealing with pride or prideful behavior. Pride prevents us from having a proper relationship with the Lord. When we believe our wisdom is better than God's, we may become a stumbling block to others. Pride destroys people with words; it causes envy, strife, divisiveness, manipulation, and evil suspicions. God detests pride and resists the proud.

You adulterous people! Do you not know that friendship with the world is enmity with God? Therefore whoever wishes to be a friend of the world makes himself an enemy of God... Therefore it says, "God opposes the proud but gives grace to the humble." Submit yourselves therefore to God. Resist the devil, and he will flee from you. Draw near to God, and he will draw near to you. (James 4:4 – 6)

Do nothing from selfish ambition or conceit, but in humility count others more significant than yourselves. Let each of you look not only to his own interests, but also to the interests of others. (Philippians 2:3 – 4)

When pride comes, then comes disgrace, but with the humble is wisdom. (Proverbs 11:2)

Do you see a man who is wise in his own eyes? There is more hope for a fool than for him. (Proverbs. 26:12)

Questions to Ponder

5.1) Consider all the expressions of pride mentioned in this lesson. In what ways are you prideful?

5.2) Pray about surrender and pride. Is there something God is asking you to surrender?

5.3) Why does He want you to surrender this?

5.4) When we surrender something, we replace it with something else. With what are you replacing the things you have surrendered? How do you fill the empty places in your life?

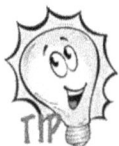

When we surrender something to the Lord, give up a harmful sin, or change a way of thinking, we may experience loss that leaves an empty place in our heart. God does not want that for us. He wants us to have joy! Surrender requires refilling!

Any gaps in your heart will be filled with something, so allow the Lord to fill those places. Seek His presence, read His Word, worship, and pray. A solid relationship with the Lord will begin to remove the loss or grief experienced from changes in our life.

Lesson 6 — Giving Up

It All Works Together

Throughout your journey, you will continue to find areas of denial, pride, and control that need to be surrendered to the Lord. Now that you understand how to identify them, it will be easier to give issues to God as they come up. Each evening, as you journal about your day, think about how control and pride are evident in your life.

What Is Surrender, and How Do I Do it?

Surrender is giving up control, laying down your pride, and being obedient to the Lord. It is vital for your journey. It sacrifices your selfish desires and changes your heart to accept God's will as your own. Surrender is coming to the end of self-effort and giving up. **It is giving up your time, will, emotions, and life to the Lord.** God wants us to live in **a state of constant surrender** to Him, a constant state of giving up to Him so He can direct our every step.

> *I know, O Lord, that the way of man is not in himself,*
> *that it is not in man who walks to direct his steps. (Jeremiah 10:23)*

We are to deny our own desires and will for His.

> *And he said to all, "If anyone would come after me, let him deny himself and take up*
> *his cross daily and follow me. For whoever would save his life will lose it, but*
> *whoever loses his life for my sake will save it." (Luke 9:23 – 24)*

How Do We Surrender?

We are promised increase when we first seek God's Kingdom, His ways, and right standing with Him. We must also abide in Him. This means we live in Him and His Spirit lives in us. Without Him, we can do nothing, but in Him we can do all things. If your first priority is to seek His kingdom, you will have all that you need.

> *But seek first the kingdom of God and his righteousness, and all these things*
> *will be added to you. (Matthew 6:33)*

> *Abide in me, and I in you. As the branch cannot bear fruit by itself, unless it abides in the*
> *vine, neither can you, unless you abide in me. I am the vine; you are the branches. Whoever*
> *abides in me and I in him, he it is that bears much fruit, for apart from me you can do*
> *nothing. If anyone does not abide in me he is thrown away like a branch and withers; and*
> *the branches are gathered, thrown into the fire, and burned. If you abide in me, and my*
> *words abide in you, ask whatever you wish, and it will be done for you. (John 15:4 – 7)*

Surrender is:

- To allow the Lord access into an area of your life
- To give up your own control and desire in that area
- To give the Lord permission to do with it what He wants
- To allow the Lord to control the outcome

When you surrender something to the Lord, the burden of the result rests on Him, not you!

Surrender Displayed through the Life of Moses

In the book of Exodus, God approached Moses, manifested as a burning bush.

> *"Come, I will send you to Pharaoh that you may bring my people, the children of Israel, out of Egypt." But Moses said to God, "Who am I that I should go to Pharaoh and bring the children of Israel out of Egypt?" ... Then Moses said to God, "If I come to the people of Israel and say to them, 'The God of your fathers has sent me to you'" and they ask me, 'What is his name?' what shall I say to them?" God said to Moses, "I AM WHO I AM." And he said, "Say this to the people of Israel: 'I AM has sent me to you."*
> *(Exodus 3:10 – 11, 13 – 14)*

Moses asked who he was to serve, and then who God was. God answered, "I AM WHO I AM." It was never about Moses or his ability to serve; **it was about God**. We do not need to be in control, because God is. **In fact, there cannot be two "I AMs" in control.** You cannot say, "I am in control of my life" and also say, "The I AM is in control of my life." One must yield. Will you keep a tight hold on your control, or give control over to the Lord?

How Do I Know What Needs to Be Surrendered? What if I Am in Denial?

One way to identify what you need to give up is to look at the causes of your anger. At times, anger is justified; many times, however, anger is an indicator of a larger issue. For instance, conversation topics that are "off-limits" because you fear how you may respond may indicate denial or something you have not fully surrendered. Sometimes we cannot understand why we do what we do. It is easier to see from an outside perspective. You may need to ask your coach, accountability partner, or **someone you respect** for his or her perspective and be **willing to hear it with an open mind**.

> ### Questions to Ponder
> 6.1) In what ways have you tried to control the outcome of situations?
>
> 6.2) What did you compromise or lose to achieve that outcome?
>
> 6.3) What things do people say or do to make you feel defensive? What life circumstances put you on the defensive?
>
> 6.4) What are the things people say or do that make you angry? What life circumstances make you angry?
>
> 6.5) What topics are not open for discussion with you? Can you spot areas in your life where being angry or threatened show something you should surrender?

Lesson 7 — Trust

Surrender Requires Trust

When we place more faith and trust in ourselves than in our God, we do not feel safe to surrender. **Trust is the crucial element that makes surrender possible** and allows a heart change. At first, trusting is difficult, but the Lord knows this and makes a way. Give Him your mustard seed of trust and watch God make it grow. Some tough situations can leave us wondering where God is. Our faith shows us that He is, in fact, there. God's Word says that He will never leave us. Just because you cannot see how He is working doesn't mean that He isn't.

Cast your burden on the LORD, and he will sustain you;
he will never permit the righteous to be moved. (Psalm 55:22)

When we become distracted, we move away from the Lord. Fear and anger make it difficult to see His work. Even when we cannot experience His presence, however, He is there. He grieves over the things that break our hearts. He sees our struggles, pain, wrong thinking, and discouragement, and He is always working in the background. The enemy makes plans to destroy us, but every time God turns them for our good. You can count on this truth.

As for you, you meant evil against me, but God meant it for good, to bring it about that many people should be kept alive, as they are today. (Genesis 50:20)

The Result of Faith and Surrender Is a Transformed Heart and Changed Life

Surrender allows God to work. He is the one who changes our hearts, gives us increase, and takes us from one measure of glory to the next. This lifelong process promises the result that we will be complete and whole.

And we all, with unveiled face, beholding the glory of the Lord, are being transformed into the same image from one degree of glory to another. For this comes from the Lord who is the Spirit.
(2 Corinthians 3:18)

And let steadfastness have its full effect, that you may be perfect and complete, lacking in nothing.
(James 1:4)

And I am sure of this, that he who began a good work in you will bring it to completion at the day of Jesus Christ. (Philippians 1:6)

And have put on the new self, which is being renewed in knowledge after the image of its creator. (Colossians 3:10)

> (!) Can you extend trust to God just for today?
>
> **Allow Him to prove Himself faithful to you.**
>
> # He will!
>
> **Then tomorrow, do it again!**
>
> You will begin growing in an unshakable faith in the Lord!

Here is how God changes our hearts:

- We believe God will save us and change our lives.

- We offer God our trust in a difficult situation.

- God proves himself trustworthy.

- We trust God over and over, and He proves His faithfulness, increasing our faith and trust in Him.

- We love God because He loves us.

- Our love transforms our desires to become more like what He desires.

- We cry out, asking Him to change what we cannot change.

- We allow God in, and then He changes our hearts and our lives. (He will not come in without our permission. We have a free will to choose His ways!)

How Do You Overcome Fear to Trust?

Imagine a mother whose teenage daughter is an addict. Even when the girl is clean, Mom cannot trust she will not lie or steal from her. This is what she has always done. She gets clean for a while, a month, maybe a year, and then it begins again. The lying starts. Mom does not know where her daughter is or what she is doing, and she is terrified she will find her daughter dead one day. Then Mom's good jewelry goes missing, along with money from her purse. The girl gets help and tries life again, but eventually fails, and the cycle begins again. It has been the same story for years.

This time, however, is different. The daughter is making an honest effort and trying hard to earn trust again, but how can her mom ever trust her? Yet if her mom never gives her trust, then she can never overcome. Her failure will always condemn her. She will never rise above her "addict" label, but Mom is afraid to trust. She cannot cope with the pain and fear of losing her daughter.

1 Corinthians 13 equates love with trusting (believing). Trust is a sacrifice.
It is a genuine act of love to allow yourself to become vulnerable.

This time, Mom does something different, too. She chooses to tell her daughter that today she will extend trust to her and see what happens. The daughter proves herself trustworthy, and Mom is pleased. Each day, she extends that gift of trust to her daughter, and each day she grows more confident in her. Eventually, she will no longer worry about her daughter failing. By trusting her daughter, Mom gives her the encouragement she needs to continue trying and doing right.

The secret is offering trust even when you believe the person, or even God, may fail you, and giving them the opportunity to prove they are trustworthy. **Trust is a gift of redemption.**

Note: There are times when it is not recommended to extend trust. You do not know if someone is ready to change their life, but God does! Listen for His wisdom. Ask your coach for additional resources.

Without the opportunity to fail, there is no opportunity to succeed.

Questions to Ponder

7.1) What places in your life do you now trust to hand over to God?

7.2) Is there a time in your life where God failed you? What happened? Whose choices were responsible for what happened?

7.3) Write *every time* you can remember in which God has been there for you, encouraged you or given you strength to get through an impossible situation.

7.4) Are you angry with God? Why?

7.5) Are you willing to give God a chance to prove Himself trustworthy to you?

Work with your coach to seek answers regarding your anger or disappointment with God.

Chapter Four

God's Expectations & Commitment

Lesson 8 — Broken Expectations

Questions to Ponder

8.1) We all have expectations of God. What do you expect of Him?

When God Disappoints Our Expectations

God tells us what we can expect from Him when we follow His ways. He will never let us down and never leave us. He meets us where we are. All He asks in return is our trust (faith) and a heart surrendered, seeking truth, willing to examine flaws, and open to being changed. God always has our best interests in mind, even if it does not always feel that way.

Misconceptions about God cause wrong expectations that lead to disappointment. When we lean too much on one characteristic of God or one part of Scripture, misunderstandings will happen. For example, if you lean too much on God's grace and ignore repentance, you may feel abandoned when you suffer the natural consequence of your sin. Likewise, if you lean too much on your works and service, you may miss relationship with God. The truth becomes skewed when we do not see the entire picture. Clarification comes when we consider the whole counsel of God's word.

If you draw two perfectly parallel lines on a piece of paper, you could continue the lines out forever, and they will never get farther apart. What if, instead, when you started to draw those lines, you were off by 0.01°? To the naked eye, the lines would appear to be parallel. As the lines are drawn out, however, they would get farther and farther away from each other. Apply this same concept to the Word of God. A small misunderstanding at the beginning can drive you further away until the truth is unrecognizable. This is why it is vital to understand how all of Scripture works together to show one complete truth.

Our Expectations of God

How do you know if your expectations of God are wrong? How do you respond when your prayers are not answered the way you expect? What happens when your faith is shaken? These questions can help identify what you are expecting from God. When God's answers seem unfair, we can find our faith shaken. Then one of three things happens:

1) **We doubt God's word.** Some people completely reject God because they feel He "didn't come through" or "allowed them to be hurt."

2) **We assume we have done something wrong that prevents God from helping us.** We sin too much or believe too little. Either way, this thinking leads to the same place: a belief that "I am not enough."

3) **We know God is good and wants what is best for us**, so there must be something **we missed or cannot yet see.** This is a good place to be. This understanding allows us to seek the Lord for answers and be patient for His response.

God Has Expectations of Us

God's plan to heal is taking away our sins and giving us new life in Him. It begins with our confession of faith, the blood of Jesus removing our sin. Then the process of **transformation into new life begins as we develop a relationship with God**. This process involves more than knowing the Scripture. It includes applying the Word of God in our lives. It is allowing the Lord into the dark places of our hearts to root out the damage, so we can put on a new identity in Him. This process requires surrender, since the Lord will not take what we will not freely give. Relationship is reciprocal, meaning that each person gives and receives from the other. Our healing is a cooperative effort with God. He has expectations of His people.

What are God's expectations? God expects that we:

- Trust and surrender control, giving the Lord permission to work in our heart

- Look at current and past situations with God's perspective

- Learn God's Word, pray, seek a relationship with Him, love Him, and listen to Him

- Pull the walls down from around our heart

- Examine our heart and remove character flaws that displease the Lord

- Put off our old self, old ways, old desires, and our past

- Guard our thoughts and make them obedient to Christ and His truth

- Share the hope we find in Jesus with others

Now this I say and testify in the Lord, that you must no longer walk as the Gentiles do, in the futility of their minds. They are darkened in their understanding, alienated from the life of God because of the ignorance that is in them, due to their hardness of heart. They have become callous and have given themselves up to sensuality, greedy to practice every kind of impurity. But that is not the way you learned Christ!—assuming that you have heard about him and were taught in him, as the truth is in Jesus, to put off your old self, which belongs to your former manner of life and is corrupt through deceitful desires, and to be renewed in the spirit of your minds, and to put on the new self, created after the likeness of God in true righteousness and holiness.
(Ephesians 4:17 – 24)

Questions to Ponder

8.2) In the past or present, what beliefs seem to have failed you?

8.3) Are your answers to question 8.2 based in truth? Search the Scripture to discover the truth according to God's word.

8.4) Are all your expectations of God reasonable? Why or why not?

8.5) Reread the list of expectations God has of us. Which expectations do you meet?

8.6) Do you object to, neglect, or misunderstand any of God's expectations?

Lesson 9 — Expect Transformation

You Can Expect a Transformed, New Life!

Count it all joy, my brothers, when you meet trials of various kinds, for you know that the testing of your faith produces steadfastness. And let steadfastness have its full effect, that you may be perfect and complete, lacking in nothing. (James 1:2 – 4)

You can expect a journey with God to transform your life into a better life in Christ. You probably believe Antarctica exists even though you have never been there to see it, yet that belief doesn't change your life. But the result of a belief in Jesus is a transformed life. The proof of transformation is the fruit demonstrated in a person's life (see Matthew 7:16). This fruit is not simply moral behavior but transformed character: love, joy, self-control, patience, kindness, goodness, gentleness, faithfulness, and peace. God's spirit is evident in a transformed heart, but transformation is a process.

We know that our old self was crucified with him in order that the body of sin might be brought to nothing, so that we would no longer be enslaved to sin. For one who has died has been set free from sin. Now if we have died with Christ, we believe that we will also live with him. (Romans 6:6 – 8)

You Can Expect Help

You can call on the Lord to help you with anything you face. He is your healer, counselor, and protector. He helps you grow spiritually. He increases your faith, teaches you His truth, and convicts you of wrong.

So we can confidently say, "The Lord is my helper; I will not fear; what can man do to me?" (Hebrews 13:6)

But the Helper, the Holy Spirit, whom the Father will send in my name, he will teach you all things and bring to your remembrance all that I have said to you. (John 14:26)

You Can Expect God to Be Patient with You

The Lord knows your beginning, your end, and all the choices you make in between. He knows the path you choose for your life, your ups and downs, and your right and wrong choices. He has great patience with you, disciplining and guiding you in gentle love to ensure your future with Him. He meets you where you are and leads you from there. You do not need to be good enough to seek God, and in fact your effort cannot make you righteous. Your sin nature corrupts your goodness so you cannot be good enough for God, but you are so valuable to God that he created a way to make you "good enough" through Christ's sacrifice.

The Lord is not slow to fulfill his promise as some count slowness, but is patient toward you, not wishing that any should perish, but that all should reach repentance. (2 Peter 3:9)

31

You Can Expect Hope, Purpose, and a Future

God has declared that His plans for you will be to your benefit. He gives you purpose, both here and in eternity. He raises you from "glory to glory" to prepare you for His plans. Your purpose on earth gives you hope and prepares you for your eternal purpose. You can trust God to help you find and fulfill that purpose.

For I know the plans I have for you, declares the Lord, plans for welfare and not for evil, to give you a future and a hope. (Jeremiah 29:11)

You Can Expect Love

As you surrender your control and fear, you become open to knowing and loving God. In return, you receive a love and acceptance from God that penetrates your heart. His love gives you confidence, approval, a sense of wellbeing, and freedom from the opinions of others.

So, we have come to know and to believe the love that God has for us. God is love, and whoever abides in love abides in God, and God abides in him. (1 John 4:16)

You Can Expect Freedom

What does freedom look like? It is abundant life in the Lord. It is casting your fear, anxiety, and worry on the Lord, lightening the load you must carry. Freedom is knowing who God is and who you are in Him. It is wielding truth to escape the guilt and shame of sin, past mistakes, and wrong choices. It is tearing down walls, discovering a new identity, and removing chains of pain and loss that keep you trapped in your own personal prison.

The Spirit of the Lord God is upon me, because the Lord has anointed me to bring good news to the poor; he has sent me to bind up the brokenhearted, to proclaim liberty to the captives, and the opening of the prison to those who are bound. (Isaiah 61:1)

So Jesus said to the Jews who had believed him, "If you abide in my word, you are truly my disciples, and you will know the truth, and the truth will set you free. … Truly, truly, I say to you, everyone who practices sin is a slave to sin. The slave does not remain in the house forever; the son remains forever. So if the Son sets you free, you will be free indeed." (John 8:31 – 32, 34 – 36)

You Can Expect God to Protect and Fight

As you begin your journey, the enemy may attack you with doubt, fear, angry thoughts, family issues, financial struggles, or anything else he can throw in your way. He will fight to keep his grip on you, but you are headed toward freedom. The Lord fights for you. A spiritual battle is taking place on your behalf. **Do not hesitate to call on God every time a situation seems too much for you to handle.** God turns every trial to your benefit. No struggle is wasted. He turns the enemy's plans against him. Be still and let God work.

No weapon that is fashioned against you shall succeed, and you shall confute every tongue that rises against you in judgment. This is the heritage of the servants of the Lord and their vindication from me, declares the Lord. (Isaiah 54:17)

The Lord will fight for you, and you have only to be silent. (Exodus 14:14)

You Can Expect Strength

When you are weak, unable to handle life, you find strength in the Lord. You find rest when you call on Him. Your weakness makes God shine. This is where He does His greatest work!

Fear not, for I am with you; be not dismayed, for I am your God; I will strengthen you, I will help you, I will uphold you with my righteous right hand. (Isaiah 41:10)

But he said to me, "My grace is sufficient for you, for my power is made perfect in weakness." Therefore I will boast all the more gladly of my weaknesses, so that the power of Christ may rest upon me. (2 Corinthians 12:9)

You Can Expect the Lord to Keep You

The Lord will not let you fall during your journey with Him. He will hold on to you and keep you on the right path when you falter. He will walk with you to the degree you allow Him, and sometimes He will even carry you. Hold Him tight, and He will keep a tight hold on you!

The Lord will keep your going out and your coming in from this time forth and forevermore. (Psalm 121:8)

Keep me as the apple of your eye; hide me in the shadow of your wings. (Psalm 17:8)

We Can Expect Relationship

When God reveals Himself to us He uses relational titles to show His desire for relationship with us. You are His beloved, His bride, His child, His friend, His servant. Relationship requires communication. Your heart speaks to Him in your prayers, and He communicates through His Spirit and written word, giving understanding and wisdom. Sometimes, He speaks through spiritual gifts. He teaches His people to hear His voice. You can expect to hear God speak.

Draw near to God, and he will draw near to you. (James 4:8a)

You Can Expect to Overcome

Nowhere does Scripture promise a trouble-free life. It says **all** will have trouble, believers and non-believers alike. The believer, however, has assurance that God is with him, and there is nothing God cannot handle. Jesus overcame the world, and in Him, you will too.

I have said these things to you, that in me you may have peace. In the world you will have tribulation. But take heart; I have overcome the world. (John 16:33)

You Can Expect Joy

Remember, there is a difference between joy and happiness. God brings you to a place where you can live in His joy. Joy is the ability not to worry or fear. When you give God your problems, pain, and fears, His joy penetrates your heart.

So also you have sorrow now, but I will see you again, and your hearts will rejoice, and no one will take your joy from you. (John 16:22)

You Can Expect Perfect Peace

Peace directly results from trust, and trust comes as you keep your mind on God's protection and provision. Knowing God takes care of you, regardless of how it seems, brings perfect peace.

You keep him in perfect peace whose mind is stayed on you, because he trusts in you.
(Isaiah 26:3)

We Can Expect a Heavenly Transplant

The power of God changes our heart. When our hardened heart breaks for Him, the Lord removes our stony heart and gives us a soft, pliable heart of flesh. He transforms us into His image like a caterpillar in a cocoon transforms into a new creation. Eventually, the caterpillar's struggle to break out of its walls ends, and a beautiful new life emerges. Your struggle too will end as the Lord breaks through your walls.

And I will give them one heart, and a new spirit I will put within them. I will remove the heart of stone from their flesh and give them a heart of flesh. (Ezekiel 11:19)

Do not love the world or the things in the world. If anyone loves the world, the love of the Father is not in him. (1 John 2:15)

Questions to Ponder

9.1) According to the Scripture passages above, what results can you expect on this journey?

9.2) Which expectations mentioned in this chapter have you experienced with God?

9.3) Has God ever disappointed you by failing to meet a "reasonable" expectation?

9.4) Why has God not always answered your expectations as you wanted?

9.5) Our free will and the free will of others can become an obstacle to our recovery. Are you willing to surrender your will for the will of God with patience for His work to come to completion?

Your faith in His word (Jesus) activates the desire in God to act in your life, and your surrender activates God's power to act. As you overcome and see His awesome works, your desires change. You will likely long to learn more about Him and His ways. The more you see Him, the more you fall in love with Him. The more you love Him, the more obedient you become. The more you seek, the more He draws near. The more He draws near, the more you look like Him!

Do not forget to write in your journal and Spend some quiet time with the Lord.

(Continue to Commitment)

Commitment

It is important to stay committed to your journey. If you give up, you will remain stuck and may even spiral into a deeper mess. It is also vital that you make a commitment to the Lord. This journey can only be taken hand-in-hand with Him. Only God can remove the damage caused by your sins and mistakes. Only He can heal your pain and set you free to be the person He created you to be.

If you have never asked God to become your Lord and save you from your sins, would you like to do that now? Do you believe in Jesus and trust Him (faith)? Are you willing to let Him be Lord in your life (willing to surrender to His will)?

What is my commitment when I invite Jesus into my life?

You are committing to relationship with the Lord. He requires your faith. He expects you to turn to Him, listening for the Holy Spirit to teach you, so you can know God (and yourself) better. He expects you to live for Him, not for the approval of man, and to learn His voice.

He wants you to surrender to His ways, (obey) and seek after Him with all your heart. He rewards those who do this with promise after promise in Scripture. Ask Him to search your heart and show you any wicked way in you. He expects your prayers and gratitude for current and future blessings.

Most importantly, He wants you to love Him!

> **If you are ready … all you need to do is tell Him!**
>
> Pray from your heart. **_To receive it, you must believe it!_** There is no specific "Sinner's Prayer" to <u>receive salvation</u>, but there are some things that you should include as you pray:
>
> - Ask forgiveness for your sins.
> - Claim your belief that Jesus is the Messiah who died to carry the burden of all your sins, and then He rose again.
> - Trust Him to lead your life in the way you should go.
> - Ask Him to become Lord of your life and invite His Spirit to live in your heart.

"And without faith it is impossible to please him, for whoever would draw near to God must believe that he exists and that he rewards those who seek him." **(Hebrews 11:6)**

"Blessed is the man who remains steadfast under trial, for when he has stood the test he will receive the crown of life, which God has promised to those who love him." (James 1:12)

"You will seek me and find me, when you seek me with all your heart." (Jeremiah 29:13)

"Search me, O God, and know my heart! Try me and know my thoughts! And see if there be any grievous way in me, and lead me in the way everlasting!" (Psalm 139:23 – 24)

"For am I now seeking the approval of man, or of God? Or am I trying to please man? If I were still trying to please man, I would not be a servant of Christ." (Galatians 1:10)

35

Introduction to Book Two

Relationship with Self

Do you struggle constantly to believe in your ability or worth? Do you despise yourself when you lose control? Is anger a perpetual war in your heart? As life goes on, we often flip-flop between confidence and doubt. Can you imagine how freeing it might be to appreciate who you are and have confidence that you will respond well to life's challenges?

You are worthy of everything God has for you because He has made you worthy!

To have confidence in yourself, you need to know yourself. To have confidence in what God can or will do in you, you need to know who God says you are in Him. Know God. Know yourself.

Don't ask yourself if you are able, but if you believe God can make you able!

In This Book

Heart Check & Inventory
You will examine the condition of your heart using methods revealed in Scripture, and you will make an inventory of your life, revealing patterns that may expose the root of your problems.

Problematic Thinking & Stuck Points
You will learn how to identify the ideas keeping you stuck and to change patterns of problematic thinking.

Self-control
You will discover how to overcome overwhelming emotions.

Perseverance
You will learn to persevere when life seems beyond hope, even when you feel attacked from every direction.

Anger Management
You will discover strategies for controlling out-of-control anger and learn the difference between destructive and beneficial anger.

Anxiety & Fear Management
Fear manifests many ways. It is the greatest tool in the enemy's arsenal. You will learn to identify fear triggers and combat them.

Chapter Five

Heart Check & Inventory

Lesson 10 — Understanding What's Ahead

Before you begin Book Two, it's important to understand how this part of your journey will work. This is the meat of your journey—one of the most difficult and rewarding parts. This lesson explains each section of this book and the heart check exercise, which you will use throughout.

The Heart Check

The heart check helps you examine the current condition of your heart and reveals both the good and the bad things hidden within it. This helps you identify areas of denial or avoidance and brings them to light where you can deal with them. It is important to remember the purpose of the heart check is to discover problems, not fix them. **You must discover what is in your heart before change can happen!**

The Heart Check Plan

After completing all the heart checks in this book, you will review your answers to identify areas where you desire change. You will define the results you want to accomplish and set goals to achieve those results. At the end of this book, you will revisit your plan and evaluate both your progress and how your goals have changed since you began.

The Inventory

The inventory is an assessment of your life that examines your resentments, fears, and hurts, along with harm you may have caused others. The inventory worksheets will help expose patterns in your life that led to detrimental relationships and behaviors. You may continue to the lessons on coping skills while working on your inventory to help you progress. However, **do not continue to the next book until your inventory is complete.** Your coach has additional tools and activities to aid the inventory process.

Coping Skills

These lessons will help you identify and deal with obstacles you may encounter on your journey. Each lesson provides a tool or acrostic teaching about problematic thinking patterns, stuck points, perseverance, powerful emotions, and managing anger and anxiety. These coping skills will remain useful even after this journey.

> ⓘ Do not continue without a coach. Now is a good time to find a strong
> accountability partner too—one who listens, keeps you balanced,
> and gives you support.

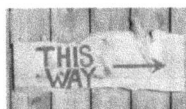

THIS WAY →	**This week, your coach will share an object lesson to illustrate the enemy's strongholds in your life and the changes that occur when you make God your only stronghold.**

Heart Check

But the Lord said to Samuel, "Do not look on his appearance or on the height of his stature, because I have rejected him. For the Lord sees not as man sees man looks on the outward appearance, but the Lord looks on the heart." (1 Samuel 16:7)

The Lord sees the genuine condition of your heart. He knows your beginning, your end, and everything in between, yet His focus is never on the outside appearance. God does not worry about the job you have, the car you drive, or the size of your body. His first concern is the state of your heart.

Every way of a man is right in his own eyes, but the Lord weighs the heart. (Proverbs 21:2)

What Is the Heart?

When God speaks about the heart, He is referring to our core being: our mind, will, and emotions. The Lord examines our desires, our motives, our plans, our schemes, and how we understand people or situations.

We hide behind layers of walls, but the Lord looks at the person beneath the layers. God knows us better than we know ourselves. He knows our wrong thoughts and actions, even those **we cannot acknowledge in ourselves but are quick to see in others**. Only with the Lord can we recognize our true condition. We lack self-control when we do not understand why we do the things we do.

For I do not understand my own actions. For I do not do what I want, but I do the very thing I hate. (Romans 7:15)

For you say, I am rich, I have prospered, and I need nothing, not realizing that you are wretched, pitiable, poor, blind, and naked. (Revelation 3:17)

Ask the Lord to test your heart and reveal needed changes. He exposes things as we become open to seeing them.

Prove me, O Lord, and try me; test my heart and my mind. (Psalm 26:2)

Create in me a clean heart, O God, and renew a right spirit within me. (Psalm 51:10)

God's word helps us understand our heart. Scripture is a mirror which reflects the condition of our character.

For the word of God is living and active, sharper than any two-edged sword, piercing to the division of soul and of spirit, of joints and of marrow, and discerning the thoughts and intentions of the heart. (Hebrews 4:12)

Question to Ponder
10.1) Do you have questions or concerns before you continue?

42

Lesson 11 — The Tongue, Part 1

One way to test your heart is by checking what comes out of your mouth. Your words are an overflow of what is in your heart. There are hundreds of scriptures regarding our words.

The good person out of the good treasure of his heart produces good, and the evil person out of his evil treasure produces evil, for out of the abundance of the heart his mouth speaks. (Luke 6:45)

But what comes out of the mouth proceeds from the heart, and this defiles a person. For out of the heart come evil thoughts, murder, adultery, sexual immorality, theft, false witness, slander. These are what defile a person. (Matthew 15:18 – 20)

It is not what goes into the mouth that defiles a person, but what comes out of the mouth; this defiles a person. (Matthew 15:11)

Read James 3

James 3 is clear that no one is innocent regarding their tongue. It is the hardest member of the body to control. This chapter compares the tongue to a blazing forest, which can set the entire course of your life on fire. Like the rudder on a ship, your will drives your speech. A tongue "set on fire by hell" is an easy tool for the enemy to use—an untamable, restless evil full of deadly poison. Believers should never spew poison; they should only give life!

Below are several scriptures that deal with the power of our words. Read the reflections and then answer the questions that follow each Scripture.

The Lord hates a deceitful and divisive mouth
Scripture mentions seven things that are an abomination to the Lord. All seven are matters of the heart, and three involve the tongue: lies, false witness, and discord.

There are six things that the Lord hates, seven that are an abomination to him: haughty eyes, a lying tongue, and hands that shed innocent blood, a heart that devises wicked plans, feet that make haste to run to evil, a false witness who breathes out lies, and one who sows discord among brothers. (Proverbs 6:16 – 19)

Question to Ponder

11.1) How often have people's words hurt you? List as many times as you can remember.

Your words are your responsibility. You must guard your tongue. Each of us will give an account **for every idle word** we speak. God is serious about our words because unchecked words cause great harm; He equates them with death. Slander and lies ruin lives. Words can destroy one's spirit, reputation, and witness. Those whose words have hurt you **will** give an account to God, and you will give an account for careless and harmful words you speak.

I tell you, on the day of judgment people will give account for every careless word they speak, for by your words you will be justified, and by your words you will be condemned.
(Matthew 12:36 – 37)

Question to Ponder

11.2) How often have your words hurt others? List as many specific instances as you can remember.

Words have the power to cause death or produce life! Our words can encourage, pray, teach, correct, witness, counsel, bless others, and honor God.

Death and <u>life</u> are in the power of the tongue, and those who love it will eat its fruits.
(Proverbs 18:21)

As Iron sharpens iron, one man sharpens another. (Proverbs 27:17)

Question to Ponder

11.3) How often have your words benefited and brought life to others? List as many specific instances as you can remember.

Guard Your Words

Whoever guards his mouth preserves his life; he who opens wide his lips comes to ruin.
(Proverbs 13:3)

How do you guard your tongue? We will not always say the right things, but we can limit the damage our tongue may cause. There is a popular saying, "We have two ears and one mouth so that we can listen twice as much as we speak." If we **are** listening, we **are not** speaking, and idle words cannot get us in trouble. Take this thought deeper. God also gave you two eyes to observe. Listening is not simply being quiet; it is seeing the meaning behind the speaker's words. Observe the speaker and ponder his words, and *your* words in response will be filled with wisdom and influence.

Listen
Listen to others before speaking and pay attention to instruction and correction.

Let every person be quick to hear, slow to speak, slow to anger. (James 1:19)

If one gives an answer before he hears, it is his folly and shame. (Proverbs. 18:13)

A fool takes no pleasure in understanding, but only in expressing his opinion. (Proverbs 18:2)

The ear that listens to life-giving reproof will dwell among the wise. (Proverbs 15:31)

The way of a fool is right in his own eyes, but a wise man listens to advice. (Proverbs 12:15)

Stop Talking

The best advice ever given: Only speak when you have something of value to say. Who gave that advice? God did. The more words you use, the more likely they will hurt someone. People place greater value on your words and message when you refrain from unnecessary speech.

Even a fool who keeps silent is considered wise; when he closes his lips, he is deemed intelligent. (Proverbs 17:28)

When words are many, sin is unavoidable, but he who restrains his lips is wise. (Proverbs 10:19)

Do you see a man who is hasty in his words? There is more hope for a fool than for him. (Proverbs 29:20)

Questions to Ponder

11.4) How well do you listen?

11.5) Do you consider the actual message someone is trying to convey, or do you seek ways to argue for your own perspective?

11.6) What changes could help you better guard your words? Commit to these changes.

Lesson 12 — The Tongue, Part 2

Gossip, Deception, and Lies, Oh My!

Has someone ever lied to you? It hurts, doesn't it? It is difficult to give trust to people capable of deceit. Lies don't just hurt our feelings; they destroy lives. People may mislead your thoughts or deceive you to act in ways you otherwise would not. They can take advantage of you, manipulate you, destroy your reputation, and involve you in legal disputes.

Deception takes many forms, from a blatant lie to subtle manipulation. It may present itself as a joke or a mistake. Deception disguised as kindness and flattery appeals to the ego while urging certain actions. Flattery is dangerous because it can manipulate you to act badly while feeling great.

Have you ever lied about your opinion of someone to protect his or her feelings? Your lie may lead others to have unreasonably high expectations, or it could cause them to feel shame and rejection. Pretending to be a friend while hiding your true feelings is deceptive and harmful.

Like a madman who throws firebrands, arrows, and death is the man who deceives his neighbor and says, 'I am only joking!' (Proverbs 26:18 – 19)

For such persons do not serve our Lord Christ, but their own appetites, and by smooth talk and flattery they deceive the hearts of the naive. (Romans 16:18)

The one who conceals hatred has lying lips, and whoever utters slander is a fool. (Proverbs 10:18)

His speech was smooth as butter, yet war was in his heart; his words were softer than oil, yet they were drawn swords. (Psalm 5521)

Keep your tongue from evil and your lips from speaking deceit. (Psalm 34:13)

Questions to Ponder

12.1) Has anyone ever lied to you? How did their lies harm you?

12.2) Have you ever lied to anyone? What harm was caused to others by your lies? (Play this lie all the way out. Who may have been hurt beyond the person you lied to? What were the unintended consequences of your lie?)

Gossip and Malicious Words

Gossip is when lies or exaggerated truth are spoken **to** us or **about** us. It could be ridicule, sharing someone's personal information, or talking about a person's mistakes or flaws. In any situation, gossip unfairly influences other's opinions about an individual.

People frequently conceal gossip as concern or a prayer request. It may be hidden in a "warning" about someone. A person may justify gossip because the hearer of the gossip is aware of the situation. They may claim it is acceptable to discuss it because it is "common knowledge". However, **the further from the source information travels, the less truth is conveyed**. The truth is often contrary to an individual's perception of a situation.

No one wants another to share their business. It is the individual's choice to share information about their lives. The choice does not belong to another.

Gossip may not start with malicious intent. It may be genuine concern for someone, legitimate prayer needs, or a simple comment relating to another's experience. You may possess a genuine belief it was an acceptable topic to discuss. Get permission before sharing anything about an individual with another person.

> Every time you share anything <u>about someone who is not you</u>, your words have the potential to become twisted and misconstrued, and to spread.

You Are Responsible

What if you do not spread gossip, but surround yourself with people who do? Just as **you are accountable for your words** and those to whom you speak them, **you are also responsible for the gossip you hear**. Every word you let into your mind influences you. Listening to someone speak about another, whether it puts them in a positive or negative light, influences your opinion of them. Hearing a false understanding or perspective can turn you against a quality person, or toward believing a deceptive one. Gossip skews truth. You are not missing out if you refuse to listen to gossip.

An evildoer listens to wicked lips, and a liar gives ear to a mischievous tongue.
(Proverbs 17:4)

Questions to Ponder

12.3) What gossip and lies have harmed you?

12.4) When did you listen to gossip and with whom?

12.5) Have you ever spread gossip and lies to others?

12.6) Have you ever shared information with an uninvolved party out of concern, or warned someone about another person? Was this gossip?

The Appeal of Juicy Morsels of Gossip

The words of a whisperer are like delicious morsels;
they go down into the inner parts of the body. (Proverbs 18:8 and 26:22)

The book of Proverbs talks twice about how appealing whispered words (i.e., gossip) are to those who listen. Gossip sinks into the inner parts of our body. The lure of gossip comes from knowing information that others do not, giving us a sense of importance. It can make us feel better about ourselves to talk about another's problems, but whenever we gossip, we are ingesting poison into the core of our soul.

12.7) How do you relate to these verses from Proverbs?

12.8) Wrong words can backfire and hurt us. Has this ever happened to you?
Describe what happened.

What if I Need to Be Advised?

Is it gossip to share with a therapist, pastor, or coach?

There is nothing wrong with seeking advice about a situation in your life that involves other people. The problem comes when you seek advice with an ill motive, or when you seek advice from those who will spread your concern to others. Seek counsel from a trusted friend—one who is fair-minded, understands your strongholds, is not afraid to call out your errors, and will offer you a realistic perspective. You can also ask for advice while keeping the person you're talking about anonymous.

If you solicit the viewpoint of someone you know will always agree with you or popular opinion, you are not requesting advice. Instead, you are venting frustration or seeking to justify yourself, and this is gossip.

Where there is no guidance, a people falls,
but in an abundance of counselors there is safety. (Proverbs 11:14)

Therapists, pastors, sponsors, and coaches should carry no bias toward you or your situation. You should feel safe to share concerns with these people, but no one is perfect. If your most trusted advisors betray your confidence, it is they who are gossiping, not you.

Watch Your Words

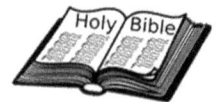

- *"A man who bears false witness against his neighbor is like a war club, or a sword, or a sharp arrow." (Proverbs 25:18)*

- *"A dishonest man spreads strife, and a whisperer separates close friends." (Proverbs 16:28)*

- *"You shall not spread a false report. You shall not join hands with a wicked man to be a malicious witness." (Exodus 23:1)*

- *"You shall not go around as a slanderer among your people, and you shall not stand up against the life of your neighbor: I am the Lord." (Leviticus 19:16)*

- *"Whoever slanders his neighbor secretly I will destroy. Whoever has a haughty look and an arrogant heart I will not endure." (Psalm 101:5)*

Sometimes we do not realize how words we speak come across to others. Pay extra close attention to your words and how people respond to them. Journal what you learn!

Lesson 13 — The Tongue, Part 3

Dealing with People Properly

How do you show love to someone who has hurt or upset you? If possible, you cover over the offense. Go directly to the person in love and help him understand his offense instead of telling others how you were mistreated. Give someone who has offended you the opportunity to make it right.

What if it were you? Would you rather be informed directly if someone has a complaint against you? Would you appreciate it if the person revealed your problem to his friends without ever addressing the issue with you?

People often evade an issue to avoid **conflict**. Avoiding the problem or venting to friends seems easier than coping with the situation. It's easy to believe that once you can "get over it," you can move on, ignoring the problem and never needing to admit your feelings to the one who wronged you. You might avoid conflict, but you do not satisfy your need for justice. As a result, animosity begins to fester.

*Whoever covers an offense seeks love, but he who repeats a matter separates close friends. (*Proverbs 17:9*)*

Whoever belittles his neighbor lacks sense, but a man of understanding remains silent. Whoever goes about slandering reveals secrets, but he who is trustworthy in spirit keeps a thing covered. (Proverbs 11:12 – 13)

Question to Ponder

13.1) In your experience, what resulted from avoiding conflict?

Conflict

Conflict is beneficial. Without conflict, restoration never happens. Burying a problem creates a larger issue. Over time, pain caused by unresolved offenses turns into anger and resentment.

Conflict resolution is not fighting. People may fear confrontation because they did not learn to engage in effective conflict, modeled in grace and love. Instead, they witnessed disputes handled through argument, belligerence, or brawling. People with shame and insecurity may also avoid conflict, fearing rejection.

Questions to Ponder

13.2) Have you ever seen healthy conflict resolution? What did it look like?

13.3) How do *you* deal with conflict?

Successful Conflict

It may seem easier to ignore an issue than deal with it, but **a person cannot fix what they do not know is broken**. The easiest and shortest way through an issue is straight ahead. A simple misunderstanding may feel like a major issue until it is addressed. But big problems are quickly solved when those involved can openly and humbly seek resolution. Incorrect handling of a situation (whether that be ignoring it, retaliation, or gossip) compounds the problem.

The Bible teaches us to engage in successful conflict.

1. Search your heart before making a judgment about another person. What angered you? Is a belief or stronghold skewing your perspective of the situation?

    Judge not, that you be not judged. For with the judgment you pronounce you will be judged, and with the measure you use it will be measured to you. (Matthew 7:1 – 2)

2. Talk about your frustration directly with the person involved, not a third party.

    If your brother sins against you, go and tell him his fault, between you and him alone. If he listens to you, you have gained your brother. (Matthew 18:15)

3. Go to the person who has offended you immediately. Don't put it off until later. God wants unresolved conflict handled first, even before giving an offering. Solving problems with others is part of a right relationship with God.

    Be angry and do not sin; do not let the sun go down on your anger, and give no opportunity to the devil. (Ephesians 4:26 – 27)

    So, if you are offering your gift at the altar and there remember that your brother has something against you, leave your gift there before the altar and go. First be reconciled to your brother, and then come and offer your gift. (Matthew 5:23 – 24)

Sowing Discord

You sow discord when, due to your actions or words, a group of people distrust one another, argue, and fight. A person who sows discord plants seeds of discontentment, making others miserable with pessimistic, hateful, or negative attitudes and leading to strife, arguing, and choosing sides.

With perverted heart devises evil, continually sowing discord. (Proverbs 6:14)

> ### Questions to Ponder
> 13.4) Do your pessimistic, negative attitudes prevent you from hearing others or seeking resolution to a problem? In what other ways do you sow discord?
>
> 13.5) In what ways do you strive to make peace?

What If You Cannot Reconcile?

What if someone refuses to hear your grievance or accept your apology? The Scripture says, "As far as it depends on you, live at peace." All you can do is make an honest effort. Do not seek vengeance. God deals with your enemies and can cause your enemies to bless you!

Repay no one evil for evil, but give thought to do what is honorable in the sight of all. If possible, so far as it depends on you, live peaceably with all. Beloved, never avenge yourselves, but leave it to the wrath of God, for it is written, "Vengeance is mine, I will repay, says the Lord."
(Romans 12:17 – 19)

When a man's ways please the Lord, he makes even his enemies to be at peace with him.
(Proverbs 16:7)

Questions to Ponder

13.6) According to the Bible, how should you handle disputes? Will it be easier this way? Why or why not?

13.7) Have you ever solved conflict using these biblical steps? What was the result?

13.8) Has anyone attempted to resolve an issue with you as described in Scripture? How did you respond? Was the situation resolved?

13.9) Are you currently holding anything against someone that needs to be addressed?

13.10) Has anyone ever rejected your efforts to resolve conflict? What was the result?

13.11) What do you consider the most challenging part of handling conflict biblically?

Lesson 14 — The Tongue, Part 4

Inappropriate and Appropriate Talk

Scripture mentions several inappropriate ways in which we use our mouths. One is dirty humor and crude comments. When we are flowing from God's Spirit, we speak what is right. When living out of our flesh, however, we speak harsh words, swear, argue, quarrel, gossip, lie, and so on. Guard your tongue! **Defer your thoughts** to the Lord before speaking. Let His Spirit show you **when to speak** and **when to be silent**.

Let there be no filthiness nor foolish talk nor crude joking, which are out of place, but instead let there be thanksgiving. (Ephesians 5:4)

But now you must put them all away: anger, wrath, malice, slander, and obscene talk from your mouth. (Colossians 3:8)

The lips of the righteous know what is acceptable, but the mouth of the wicked, what is perverse. (Proverbs 10:32)

What Should You Say?

- Use words that are appropriate and full of grace.
  "Let no corrupting talk come out of your mouths, but only such as is good for building up, as fits the occasion, that it may give grace to those who hear." (Ephesians 4:29)

- Your speech should preserve what is good and right, like salt preserves meat. You should give answers full of grace and love, not wrath.
  "Let your speech always be gracious, seasoned with salt, so that you may know how you ought to answer each person." (Colossians 4:6)

- Discuss what is fitting to encourage and help others.
  "A word fitly spoken is like apples of gold in a setting of silver." (Proverbs 25:11)

- Encourage and build up others with your words.
  "Therefore encourage one another and build one another up, just as you are doing." (1 Thessalonians 5:11)

- Give straightforward, honest, yes or no answers.
  "But above all, my brothers, do not swear, either by heaven or by earth or by any other oath, but let your "yes" be yes and your "no" be no, so that you may not fall under condemnation." (James 5:12)

- Pray with gratitude and thanksgiving. Make intercessions for others to lead godly lives.
  "First of all, then, I urge that supplications, prayers, intercessions, and thanksgivings be made for all people, for kings and all who are in high positions, that we may lead a peaceful and quiet life, godly and dignified in every way." (1 Timothy 2:1 – 15)

- Speak truth. *"Therefore, having put away falsehood, let each one of you speak the truth with his neighbor, for we are members one of another."* (Ephesians 4:25)

- Praise others, not yourself. *"Let another praise you, and not your own mouth; a stranger, and not your own lips."* (Proverbs 27:2)

14.1) What circumstances cause you to struggle with inappropriate words?

14.2) How well do you use life-giving words? Can you improve?

Consequences of the Tongue

- *"You shall not take the name of the Lord your God in vain, <u>for the Lord will not hold him guiltless</u> who takes his name in vain. (Exodus 20:7)*

- *"Remind them of these things and charge them before God not to quarrel about words, which does no good, but <u>only ruins the hearers.</u>" (2 Timothy 2:14)*

- *"There is one whose <u>rash words are like sword thrusts</u>, but the tongue of the wise brings healing." (Proverbs 12:18)*

- *"A soft answer turns away wrath, but <u>a harsh word</u> <u>stirs up anger.</u>" (Proverbs 15:1)*

- *"A gentle tongue is a tree of life, but <u>perverseness</u> in it <u>breaks the spirit.</u>" (Proverbs 15:4)*

- *"The words of a wise man's mouth win him favor, but the <u>lips of a fool consume him.</u> The beginning of the words of his mouth is foolishness, and the end of his talk is <u>evil madness.</u>" (Ecclesiastes 10:12-13)*

- *"The lips of the righteous feed many, but <u>fools die for lack of sense.</u>" (Proverbs 10:21)*

- *"If anyone thinks he is religious and <u>does not bridle his tongue</u> but <u>deceives his heart,</u> this person's <u>religion is worthless.</u>" (James 1:26)*

Congratulations!
You have completed the heart check on the tongue!

Questions to Ponder

14.3) Review your answers from all the lessons on the tongue and write down anything you do well.

14.4) Write about any areas discussed in the lessons on the tongue where you need to improve.

14.5) How do you feel about this heart check?

Lesson 15 — Your Thoughts, Part 1

Test Your Heart by Knowing Your Thoughts

You can test your heart by examining the secret thoughts you never reveal to anyone or even those thoughts you refuse to acknowledge. Thoughts invoke feelings and desires. Therefore, what we feel, think, and desire (our "will") displays the core condition of our heart.

Search me, O God, and know my heart! Try me and know my thoughts! (Psalm 139:23)

Questions to Ponder

15.1) What thoughts have you kept secret? Seek the Lord and ask Him to reveal thoughts you struggle to acknowledge or refuse to admit, even to yourself. List them to bring them into the light.

15.2) How do your secret thoughts affect your life? (Consider your emotions, actions, etc.)

Renew Your Mind

Feelings often direct our conscious thoughts. Changing our thoughts can alter the way we feel and what we desire. Different thinking can override negative emotions. Science has shown that, as our thinking changes, the make-up of our brain changes. The renewal of the mind spoken of in Scripture is the process of replacing poisonous patterns of thinking.

Do not be conformed to this world, <u>but be transformed by the renewal of your mind</u>, that by testing you may discern what is the will of God, what is good and acceptable and perfect. (Romans 12:2)

God's transformation changes how we think. We hear two conflicting reports throughout our lives: lies of the enemy leading to death, or to the true report of the Lord, which leads to life. We choose which one we listen to. Believe the report of the Lord. Choose life and live!

I call heaven and earth to witness against you today, that I have set before you life and death, blessing and curse. Therefore choose life, that you and your offspring may live. (Deuteronomy 30:19)

Our minds require renewal. Without the Lord, our thoughts turn to evil and become enslaved to our flesh.

The Lord saw that the wickedness of man was great in the earth, and that <u>every intention</u> of the <u>thoughts of his heart</u> was only evil continually. (Genesis 6:5)

Therefore, we must guard our minds from the enemy's lies and wrong thinking by keeping our mind focused on the Lord. We must take our thoughts captive, controlling what we allow our mind to absorb.

Set your minds on things that are above, not on things that are on earth. (Colossians 3:2)

You keep him in perfect peace whose mind is stayed on you, because he trusts in you. (Isaiah 26:3)

We destroy speculations and every lofty thing raised up against the knowledge of God, and we take every thought captive to the obedience of Christ. (2 Corinthians 10:5)

How do you take your thoughts captive?

➢ Keep your mind focused on what is good and worthy of praise.

"Finally, brothers, whatever is true, whatever is honorable, whatever is just, whatever is pure, whatever is lovely, whatever is commendable, if there is any excellence, if there is anything worthy of praise, think about these things." (Philippians 4:8)

➢ Guard what goes into your mind. This may include videos, books, or music. Keep your eyes from wicked things that may "cling to you" or have a lasting impact.

"I will not set before my eyes anything that is worthless. I hate the work of those who fall away; it shall not cling to me. (Psalm 101:3)

➢ Set your mind on furthering God's Kingdom and seeking the will of God. Do not become preoccupied by worldly things. The priorities and motivations of this world are not the same priorities and motivations that move a person seeking after God's heart.

"But he turned and said to Peter, 'Get behind me, Satan! You are a hindrance to me. For you are not setting your mind on the things of God, but on the things of man.'"
(Matthew 16:23)

"As we look not to the things that are seen but to the things that are unseen. For the things that are seen are transient, but the things that are unseen are eternal."
(2 Corinthians 4:18)

"For to set the mind on the flesh is death, but to set the mind on the Spirit is life and peace. For the mind that is set on the flesh is hostile to God, for it does not submit to God's law; indeed, it cannot. Those who are in the flesh cannot please God."
(Romans 8:6 – 8)

➢ Do not lean on your own understanding. Instead, seek God, and He will keep you on the right path. There is no fear when we trust in the Lord. Our emotions, senses, and experiences blind us to truth when filtered through our strongholds—the protection responses created by our life experiences. We know truth by God's wise counsel.

"Trust in the Lord with all your heart, and do not lean on your own understanding. In all your ways acknowledge Him, and He will make your paths straight. Do not be wise in your own eyes." (Proverbs 3:5 – 7)

"Seek after the Lord always. With my whole heart I seek you; let me not wander from your commandments!" (Psalm 119:10)

"He is not afraid of bad news; his heart is firm, trusting in the Lord." (Psalm 112:7)

Questions to Ponder

15.3) How have you tried to take your thoughts captive in the past?

15.4) Do you base your judgments and choices on what you think happened without knowing all the facts? Give examples.

15.5) Do you tend to focus more on the positive or negative? List the ways your thoughts focus on the negative.

15.6) What impact does your negativity have on you?

15.7) For each negative thought you mentioned, how can you change to more positive thoughts?

15.8) What do you allow to influence your mind? (TV, movies, books, friends, etc.)

15.9) How do things you watch, read, and hear "cling" to you?

15.10) What should you stop watching, reading, and hearing?

Lesson 16 — Your Thoughts, Part 2

Priorities Are Thoughts That Define Our Heart

We invest in our heart's desire, but our treasure is more than monetary. We treasure time, perhaps to a greater extent than we value money. How many times have you paid extra for a timesaving convenience? Money is replaceable, but time spent is lost forever. Time is our greatest treasure.

For where your treasure is, there will your heart be also. (Luke 12:34)

To understand what your heart most values, examine how you spend your time and why. We make many plans for our time, but the Lord directs the steps of a believer. How do you manage your time? Do you stay busy and use time wisely? Is your time spent in a manner pleasing to the Lord?

Look carefully then how you walk, not as unwise. but as wise, making the best use of the time, because the days are evil. Therefore do not be foolish, but understand what the will of the Lord is. (Ephesians 5:15 – 17)

The heart of man plans his way, but the Lord establishes his steps. (Proverbs 16:9)

Questions to Ponder

16.1) **Prioritize the following list according to their importance to you.**
(1 being the most important and 14 being the least important)

___Career/School   ___Video Games

___Family   ___Social Media

___Friends   ___Prayer/Worship (*Relationship w/God*)

___Extended Family   ___Read/Study Bible

___Finances/Planning   ___House Cleaning/Yard Work

___Television/Music/Reading ___Serving others/Evangelism

___Entertainment/Dining Out ___Church Services/Functions

16.2) **We often allow unimportant things to take priority in our lives. Examine your priority list. Write the approximate time you spend with each item on the list in a typical week.**

16.3) **Is the time you spend appropriate for the priority you place on it?**

16.4) **How would God prioritize this list?**

16.5) **To which priorities should you give more or less time?**

Priorities According to the Word

God's Word clearly defines what our top priority should be: God comes first. Why is it so difficult for us Christians to give God precedence? We live in a world full of distractions that absorb our time. Our responsibilities and people's expectations constantly demand our attention. In addition, our own desires vie for our time. God does not want us to abandon our hobbies or interests, but He expects to be our first love. Is your relationship with God first on your priority list?

Consider the following scriptures and reexamine your priorities.

> *"And whatever you do, in word or deed, do everything in the name of the Lord Jesus, giving thanks to God the Father through him." (Colossians 3:17)*

> *"But seek first the kingdom of God and his righteousness, and all these things will be added to you." (Matthew 6:33)*

> *"For what does it profit a man to gain the whole world and forfeit his soul? For what can a man give in return for his soul?" (Mark 8:36 – 37)*

> *"So flee youthful passions and pursue righteousness, faith, love, and peace, along with those who call on the Lord from a pure heart." (2 Timothy 2:22)*

> *"For while bodily training is of some value, godliness is of value in every way, as it holds promise for the present life and also for the life to come." (1 Timothy 4:8)*

> *'Whoever loves father or mother more than me is not worthy of me, and whoever loves son or daughter more than me is not worthy of me." (Matthew 10:37)*

Questions to Ponder

16.6) What distractions prevent you from spending time with the Lord?

16.7) Is your focus more on worldly or heavenly things? How so?

16.8) Are you trusting God with your time? Explain.

16.9) Consider changing your priorities. How do you want your priorities to look?

Lesson 17 — Your Thoughts, Part 3

Searching Your Heart by the Word of God: The Bible Is Your Mirror

To take our thoughts captive to the obedience of Christ is to examine them in the light of God's Word. When you read the Bible, it is like looking in a mirror. As you read, Scripture exposes your thoughts and feelings, showing you the truth about yourself. In this way, **Scripture helps you know your heart as God sees it**. However, **if you are not open** to accepting the truth you find, **God's truth cannot change your life**.

For the word of God is living and active, sharper than any two-edged sword, piercing to the division of soul and of spirit, of joints and of marrow, and discerning the thoughts and intentions of the heart. (Hebrews 4:12)

Our thoughts, feelings, and actions work together to display our heart's condition. We filter messages from people, media, the internet, or other sources through our worldview.

Your **worldview** comprises your preconceived ideas about **how the world is**. Your **philosophy** is your belief about **what life should be** based on past teachings, experiences, fears, and strongholds. As if seeing the world through tinted glasses, we view new information from the perspective created by our philosophy and worldview.

Like anything else, we can filter Scripture through past teaching, our worldview, fears, and strongholds. Therefore, it is important to **ask the Lord for understanding** every time we read His Word, and to **keep an open mind to anything God wants to say**. He will show us truth, but we will derive no good from it if we refuse to listen.

Pray that God will show you the condition of your heart as you read the following passages of Scripture and consider what this means for you.

Everyone who hates his brother is a murderer, and you know that no murderer has eternal life abiding in him. (1 John 3:15)

If anyone says, "I love God," and hates his brother, he is a liar; for he who does not love his brother whom he has seen cannot love God whom he has not seen. (1 John 4:20)

Whoever says he is in the light and hates his brother is still in darkness. (1 John 2:9)

Question to Ponder

17.1) **Do you hold hatred in your heart toward another? (These passages are referring not only to a biological brother, but to another in Christ.)**

Doing wrong is like a joke to a fool, but wisdom is pleasure to a man of understanding.
(Proverbs 10:23)

Question to Ponder

17.2) Do you ever perceive something wrong as being funny? (Include things from TV, the Internet, movies, social media, and other entertainment sources.)

Love is patient and kind; love does not envy or boast; it is not arrogant or rude. It does not insist on its own way; it is not irritable or resentful. (1 Corinthians 13:4 – 5)

Questions to Ponder

17.3) When do you struggle with patience and kindness?

17.4) Do you envy anyone (desiring what they have)?

17.5) Do you boast about your possessions, your experiences, or your successes? Do you make sure other people can see your possessions or successes (boasting without words)? Explain.

17.6) Do you need to be in control or insist on getting your way? How do you do this?

17.7) What ways do you assume you know better than others?

17.8) List the causes of your irritability or resentments.

For although they knew God, they did not honor him as God or give thanks to him, but they became futile in their thinking, and their foolish hearts were darkened. (Romans 1:21)

Questions to Ponder

17.9) Consider what you grumbled or complained about today, or this week. What complaints are expressed in your words or hidden in your heart?

17.10) List everything for which you can thank God. Take a minute to tell God how thankful you are!

Complaining is a selfish behavior, focusing on a desired outcome and disregarding the reality of a situation. It is a mindset blinded to alternative possibilities. It discounts the desires or needs of others and ignores the blessings God gives in the wake of hard trials. People with a mentality bent on grumbling pay little attention to the good surrounding them. They focus on everything that is not "right" or "fair" in the world, and they discount people's good qualities, instead fixating on their flaws.

Questions to Ponder

17.11) How do you fail to notice positive things and dwell on the negative?

17.12) Consider the situations you grumble about. How are your complaints discounting God's work or nature?

And he said to him, "You shall love the Lord your God with all your heart and with all your soul and with all your mind." (Matthew 22:37)

Questions to Ponder

17.13) Do you apply the command to "love God with all your heart, mind, and soul" in your life? How would you like to do so?

Lesson 18 — Your Thoughts, Part 4

Motives

Motives are the intentions or reasons behind our choices. Sometimes we do the right thing with ill motives. Perhaps our motives are honorable, but our actions result in an unintended outcome. Many times we are unaware, or refuse to consider, the motives that dwell in our subconscious thoughts. We need to examine the motives behind our thoughts, words, actions, and even our prayers.

Thoughts and motives interlink. Our thoughts influence our motives, and our motives influence our thoughts, which direct our decisions. Thoughts and ideas filtered through fear, insecurity, selfishness, and our individual versions of right and wrong give birth to wrong, selfish motives. **Regardless of the outcome, it is the heart's intent that matters to God.** Doing good things with wicked intention is sin. And when our heart's motives line up with God's ways, mistakes resulting in a negative outcome are not always sinful. God examines the spirit in which we act. He does **not condemn** us for **honest mistakes** when we strive to be obedient to His Word.

> *Repent, therefore, of this wickedness of yours, and pray to the Lord that,*
> *if possible, the intent of your heart may be forgiven you. (Acts 8:22)*

Questions to Ponder

18.1) Define in your own words which intentions of your heart please the Lord, and which motives He would consider wickedness.

18.2) How do your motives influence your thoughts, ideas, decisions, or actions?

Influence

Be careful with whom you associate. Everything you see and hear influences your thoughts, and the people in your life are your greatest influence. Your spouse and close friendships should have similar values and beliefs to yours. It is difficult, sometimes painful, and often detrimental when your close relationships oppose your faith. Scripture calls this being **unequally yoked.**

If your friends are not of moral character, you will pick up more of their bad habits than they will pick up of your good ones. You may keep your core values, but people do affect how you think. Are you a people pleaser? Your desire for approval affects your motives. Guarding your mind includes guarding which influences you allow in.

> *Do two walk together, unless they have agreed to meet?*
> *(Amos 3:3)*

> *The fear of man lays a snare, but whoever trusts in the Lord is safe.*
> *(Proverbs 29:25)*

18.3) Do you keep company with people of godly character?

18.4) Do you compromise your values or change your behavior when with certain people?

18.5) Do you behave in certain ways to be accepted or to avoid another's judgment?

Emotions

Our emotions often speak louder than our thoughts. Thoughts are the place where our emotions dwell. Emotions develop as our minds interpret situations through our conscious thoughts, memories, and beliefs. This is how our emotions can help us understand our unconscious thoughts. **When you discover the thought behind an emotion, you discover what is in your heart, which helps you understand your expectations and sort through your motives.**

In the **conscious mind,** the part of the mind in which we are currently aware and process our thoughts, it is easy to connect a thought to the emotion it evokes. For example, if someone cuts you off in traffic, you think, "They almost caused a wreck!" and you experience fear. Your fear connects to your realization that you almost wrecked your car.

Have you ever experienced an emotion, like sadness or fear, that seems to have no origin? Thoughts buried in the **unconscious mind** can trigger an emotional response that seems illogical or out of place, like experiencing sudden fear or sadness when you step outside.

Think of your brain as a personal computer. Every thought, emotion, memory, and belief becomes a file stored on the hard drive of your brain. The **conscious mind** is like your open, active files. The **subconscious mind** is like your file storage, which gives you easy access to thoughts, knowledge, and emotions, which your conscious mind may pull up as needed.

Once the conscious mind processes a thought, it files it in a directory called memory in the **unconscious mind**. If the mind believes the thought is accurate knowledge, it stores it as a **belief**. Your brain automatically files every thought, emotion, belief, and memory. While your mind is assimilating current experiences, it is running scans of all your stored files, seeking relevant information.

If an **unconscious process** of your brain triggers an emotional response, your conscious mind will know the emotion, but it may not be aware of the reason for it. This is when **you must step back and learn what your emotions are telling you.**

Toxic Emotions or Toxic Thoughts?

Emotions **can inform you** of your thoughts, but they **should *never* guide** your decisions. Even though they generate powerful feelings, **emotions have no ability to decipher between right and wrong.** Emotions are neither good nor bad, but if they develop from strongholds and wrong thinking, they can deceive you or control you.

Not all emotions that feel bad are toxic. Grief feels bad, but the message grief portrays is deep love for another. People only grieve for what they love. **Toxic emotions are emotions that trap you or feed your flesh's sin nature, drawing you away from God or people.** Envy feeds the sin of lust or jealousy can cause dissention. Fear can be a healthy emotion that protects you from danger, or it can become toxic, crippling you from making positive changes in your life.

What determines whether an emotion is healthy or toxic, is the message or thought behind it and your response to it. For example, anger shows a real or perceived injustice; it is neither positive nor negative. However, your response to anger may be considered either good or evil. We can allow anger to fester into hate or use the information it gives us to resolve a conflict and forgive another person.

It is thoughts, not emotions, which are healthy or destructive. Therefore, it is vital to determine the truth about your thoughts. This keeps your heart in right standing with the Lord and prevents your flesh from using your emotions to trigger sin.

It may be difficult to identify the thought causing a certain emotion. Think about **what happened before you felt it. Are you feeling another emotion as well? What are you thinking now? Does this emotion feel like something you have experienced in the past?** Answering these questions can help you discover whether the feeling is rational or based on a lie.

Do not confuse thoughts with feelings. We can express feelings in one or two words, but if you need a sentence to express a feeling, you are likely sharing a thought. "I feel like I don't deserve love" is a thought, not an emotion. "I feel shame," on the other hand, expresses an emotion.

Questions to Ponder

18.6) How well do you handle your emotions? Explain.

18.7) Do you feel emotions which seem to have no cause? Explain.

18.8) Pay attention to your emotions this week. Using the questions in bold above, examine the thoughts behind each emotion. Are these toxic or healthy thoughts?

18.9) Were you unable to identify the underlying thought of an emotion? Describe the emotion and the circumstances surrounding it.

Congratulations!
You have completed the heart check on your thoughts!

Questions to Ponder

18.10) Review all your answers from the lessons on thoughts and write down any ways in which you do well.

18.11) Write about any areas discussed in the lessons on thoughts where you need to improve.

18.12) How do you feel about this heart check?

Lesson 19 — Your Actions, Part 1

Actions

Your actions show the condition of your heart. Situations lead to thoughts, which result in actions. Examine your actions to discover the feelings and thoughts that triggered the action. We must know why we behave as we do to understand and guard our hearts.

Above all else, guard your heart, for everything you do flows from it. (Proverbs 4:23)

We invest our time, money, and attention in what we treasure.

Integrity

If your words say one thing but your actions say another, you are disingenuous. Scripture says to let your words be simply "yes" or "no" (see Matthew 5:37), referring to your integrity. Your word alone should be as dependable as a vow. Consider this parable:

"But what do you think? A man had two sons. And he went to the first and said, 'Son, go and work in the vineyard today.' And he answered, 'I will not,' but afterward he changed his mind and went. And he went to the other son and said the same. And he answered, 'I go, sir,' but did not go. Which of the two did the will of his father?" They said, "The first." Jesus said to them, "Truly, I say to you, the tax collectors and the prostitutes go into the kingdom of God before you. For John came to you in the way of righteousness, and you did not believe him, but the tax collectors and the prostitutes believed him. And even when you saw it, you did not afterward change your minds and believe him."
(Matthew 21:28 – 32)

Questions to Ponder

19.1) How do the things you say differ from your genuine feelings and actions?

19.2) Do you ever give into laziness, avoid work, or make excuses?

This parable applies to every life situation. If our words say one thing but our actions say the opposite, we are not trustworthy. We see this lack of integrity in **the masks** we wear for certain people, **lies** we tell to fit in, **excuses** made to avoid work, and **claiming to** believe or like something to gain approval. In every case, our actions do not match our words or what is really in our heart. When this happens, we are not being honest.

Who is wise and understanding among you? By his good conduct let him show his works in the meekness of wisdom. But if you have bitter jealousy and selfish ambition in your hearts, do not boast and be false to the truth. This is not the wisdom that comes down from above, but is earthly, unspiritual, demonic. For where jealousy and selfish ambition exist, there will be disorder and every vile practice. But the wisdom from above is first pure, then peaceable, gentle, open to reason, full of mercy and good fruits, impartial and sincere. And a harvest of righteousness is sown in peace by those who make peace. (James 3:13 – 18)

Questions to Ponder

19.3) Jealousy and selfish ambition (seeking to acquire success at the expense of another) produce disorder and vile actions. How have your jealousy or ambition become harmful?

19.4) True wisdom comes from good motives and leads to peace, mercy, reasonableness, and other good actions. Describe the positive result of your good conduct?

So, whether you eat or drink, or whatever you do, do all to the glory of God.
(1 Corinthians 10:31)

Question to Ponder

19.5) We are told to glorify God in everything we do, even the little things! In what ways do your actions glorify God?

Scripture speaks of "numbering our days." This refers to our brief existence on earth compared to eternity. As we consider our limited number of days, we make what we do in those days count, and choose not to waste any time.

Who considers the power of your anger, and your wrath according to the fear of you?
So teach us to number our days that we may get a heart of wisdom. (Psalm 90:11 – 12)

Questions to Ponder

19.6) How much time do you spend on self-gratifying or trivial activities?

19.7) What activities do you consider a waste of time?

19.8) How do you expect the Lord wants you to use your time?

How you invest your money and possessions is a powerful statement to the condition of your heart. It displays either your love for God and people or your level of greed. God wants you to give from the genuine desire of your heart, not just because it is the "right thing to do."

Generosity goes further than giving stuff. Often the most valuable gift we can give to another is our time and our ear. Good listeners support and encourage others. Giving your time is a genuine display of love and kindness to a person and service to the Lord.

Each one must give as he has decided in his heart, not reluctantly or under compulsion,
for God loves a cheerful giver. (2 Corinthians 9:7)

Sell your possessions and give to the needy. Provide yourselves with moneybags that do not grow old, with a treasure in the heavens that does not fail, where no thief approaches and no moth destroys. For where your treasure is, there will your heart be also.
(Luke 12:33 – 34)

No servant can serve two masters, for either he will hate the one and love the other, or he will be devoted to the one and despise the other. You cannot serve God and money. (Luke 16:13)

Questions to Ponder

19.9) In what do you invest a significant amount of money?

19.10) If your spending does not represent your treasure, what changes must you make?

19.11) Do you hold your possessions with a firm grip, or are you open to giving them away if the situation calls for it? What are you unwilling to let go?

19.12) You invest your time and attention in what you treasure. Are you quick to give time to others? Why or why not?

19.13) Are you attentive when listening to others? Do you let other things—the time, your phone, or a squirrel outside—distract you?

Lesson 20 — Your Actions, Part 2

Be angry, and do not sin; ponder in your own hearts on your beds, and be silent. (Psalm 4:4)

Questions to Ponder

20.1) List all the ways your anger causes you to sin.

20.2) Do you say words you should not say, or words you regret out of anger?

20.3) How do you control your angry responses?

20.4) What makes you angry? Does your anger come because you were hurt, fearful, or desire something you cannot get? Is your anger because of an injustice?

The wise of heart will receive commandments, but a babbling fool will come to ruin.
(Proverbs 10:8)

Questions to Ponder

20.5) How well do you receive correction? Be honest: Do you place blame on others?

20.6) How do you respond to rules or when confronted?

20.7) Do you listen more than you speak? How well do you hear others?

20.8) Does your opinion matter, and to whom?

20.9) Do you talk over others or talk a lot because you feel people do not hear or value what you say?

The heart is deceitful above all things, and desperately sick; who can understand it?
"I the Lord search the heart and test the mind, to give every man according to his ways,
according to the fruit of his deeds." (Jeremiah 17:9 – 10)

Question to Ponder

20.10) Pray and ask the Lord to search your heart and test your mind and actions. What has He revealed to you?

Congratulations!
You have completed the heart check on your actions!

Questions to Ponder

20.11) Review all your answers from the actions lessons and write down any areas you do well.

20.12) Write down all areas from the action lessons where you need improvement.

20.13) How do you feel about this heart check? *(Continue to next page)*

For this people's heart has grown dull, and with their ears they can barely hear, and their eyes they have closed; lest they should see with their eyes and hear with their ears and understand with their heart and turn, and I would heal them. (Acts 28:27)

Do not be discouraged by a negative answer in your heart check. Do not worry; this does not mean you are a bad person or beyond hope. Your heart check was never intended to condemn you, but to expose areas of your flesh that hinder you. Do not be disappointed with yourself, thinking, "So much is wrong with me." Everyone has wrong thoughts and desires, and everyone acts on them sometimes. You will soon discover that those things **do not define you**.

The solution is seeking the Lord and repenting when He points out an issue. Refusing to examine or repent from an issue may harden your heart, which creates a dull, cold, miserable person. However, if you bring your flaws into the open, God removes them. Don't expect all your flaws to change at once, either; this will only overwhelm you. Transformation is a lifelong process. Give your sin to God and let Him make you into His image!

Repentance

What does it mean to repent? Repentance is not just saying you are sorry. Many people believe that if you say you are sorry and really mean it, then all is forgiven, and you can move forward. It is true, you must sincerely apologize, but repentance is not moving forward. It is turning around. It is turning from your sin to head in the opposite direction, back to God.

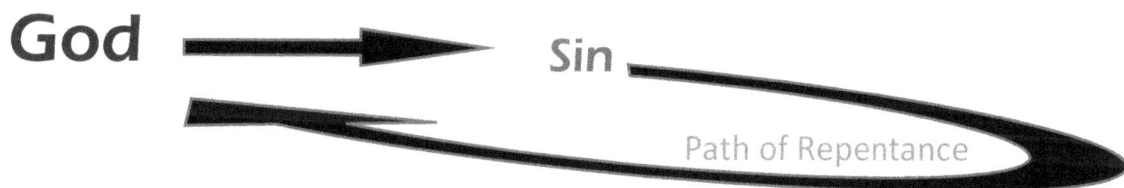

Questions to Ponder

20.14) Go back through your answers at the end of each heart check section. Write down the areas for improvement that you mentioned in each one.

20.15) Change is a process that takes time. To start that process, repent.

- Make a conscious decision to change each one of these things and ask for the Lord's forgiveness where needed.
- Pray. Tell God your desire to repent and ask Him to change your heart!
- Write what you think about your choice. Do you believe that God will change your heart as you desire?

20.16) Use the worksheet on the next page to create some goals you wish to work toward with the Lord.

Making a "Heart Check Plan"

Putting the Pieces Together

You have come a long way by recognizing the condition of your heart. Here is the good news: The areas that need improving do not define who you are! Every person has some things in their heart that need to be changed or that they wish were different. You have likely discovered some of these things in yourself. You have also seen the good in your heart, such as times you have shown compassion, used words to encourage, and so on.

What do you do with this information? The first step is to understand exactly what needs to be corrected and the person you desire to become. As your journey continues, you will discover the root of your heart issues. You will see how it is possible for the Lord to transform you into the person He created you to be, and you will learn to keep your heart in check to prevent falling back into old ways.

Directions:

List the things you wish to change, and the result you wish to see.
You may copy this page or write the lists in your journal.

List the areas you wish to change.

_____
_____
_____
_____
_____
_____
_____
_____
_____
_____
_____
_____
_____
_____
_____
_____
_____
_____

For each change, write the desired result.

_____
_____
_____
_____
_____
_____
_____
_____
_____
_____
_____
_____
_____
_____
_____
_____
_____
_____

What do you feel is (are) your most damaging issue(s)?

_____
_____
_____
_____

Questions to Ponder

20.17) Reference the "Making a Heart Check Plan" worksheet.
For each change you want to see, write a scripture that encourages you towards making that change.

- * Start by focusing on your most damaging issue.

- * Memorize the verse for the issue you are addressing.

- * When you struggle with the issue, consider the verse and journal.

- * Do not attempt to solve every issue at once. Allow the Lord to guide you.

Lesson 21 — Take Inventory of Your Life

Now that you know what is in your heart, it is time to investigate where it originated. We start life with a sin nature; that means we have a tendency toward sin. However, it is our experiences that bring about fear, anger, depression, loneliness, insecurity, shame, and so on. These are the root causes of most addictions, codependency, and destructive behaviors.

The First Step

The first step of your inventory prepares your mind to examine past hurts. For some people, the pain of their past causes blocked or denied emotions. This makes it difficult to be honest about the experiences associated with that pain. Your heart check was a good starting point. Examine your answers and find clues that show your feelings.

Invest yourself in the following questions. **Take your time and give thorough answers**. When you feel as if you have found every answer, ask yourself, "What else?" Continue to seek what else you can add until you have completely exhausted all possibilities.

> ### First Step Questions
>
> 21.1)   What things anger you? (Past experiences, loss, missed opportunities, abuse, etc.)
>
> 21.2)   What are your fears? (People, Illness, rejection, loss, failure, abandonment, opinions, the future, etc.)
>
> 21.3)   What do you feel guilty about? Why do you feel shame?
>
> 21.4)   Are you honest? Do you make excuses and feel like a victim (self-pity), or blame others for your faults?

The Second Step

Everything so far has prepared you for your inventory. This is a tremendous step toward changing the bad thinking behind the destructive behaviors and addictions that rule your life, but it can be a difficult process. Completing your inventory will help you identify the negative messages that shaped your self-image and behaviors, and teach you beneficial ways to think about your life. Thinking differently can change the impact of painful life events.

In Step Two, you will list significant events in your life. If you avoid thinking about certain times in life or have difficulty acknowledging painful words and circumstances, this step may seem overwhelming or frightening. Admitting your poor choices and the pain others have caused you can be painful and embarrassing. Do not get stuck in these feelings. Trust God and your coach to get you through.

> ➤ Realize you are safe. Your coach experienced his own situations that left similar scars on his heart. His experience may not be the same, but he understands pain and shame. Your coach will not judge or condemn you.

> ➤ Remember gratitude. Think how far you have already come. Remember all the Lord has done and trust He will never leave you. Remember that praise is the key that unlocks your freedom.

Instructions for the Step Two Worksheet

Carefully read the following instructions before beginning.

The Step Two Worksheet will guide you through your life inventory. *Remembering back as far as possible, list every significant event in your life. Be as honest and thorough as possible. Trying to remember what happened in your life can be difficult. It helps to consider your life in seasons and groups (i.e., family, school, college, marriage, significant friendships, work relationships, and so on).*

- Start by listing just the events leaving out details, messages, or emotions related to the situation.
- After completing every list on the worksheet, write causes for each item on each list.
- Then go back through your lists again and write the messages for each item on each list.

What are messages?

After writing each list (and causes), you will write the messages received from the situation you listed. A "message" is the impression left on your heart from others' words or actions (whether or not the person intended to imply the message by their words or actions). How did the situation speak into your life or about your character and worth? Hidden messages significantly influence how you view yourself.

For example: Your aunt tells you, "You are just like your father." If your father is a brilliant, moral, successful man, the message you receive would be affirming. However, if your father was a drunk and absent from your life, the unspoken message you hear might be, "I will never amount to anything" or "I am rejected, worthless." In this case, the root of the message is your opinion of your father. Your aunt may have noticed something that resembled a positive trait or talent your father has, but you hear her words filtered through your own pre-conceived ideas about him.

How to identify significant events

List people and/or situations that occurred during major life events, trials, or addiction. Include any event related to an issue you recognize. Think about the answers you wrote to the questions in Step One. What life situations are related to or impacted by those feelings? (For example, if you have an intense fear of rejection, include situations in which you felt left out or ridiculed.)

List any situation or comment that reinforced a destructive message. (For instance, someone saying you are an unwanted child seems insignificant but reinforces the message that you are not loveable.) Any comment that still sticks out in your mind is significant. You may add to your lists anytime during this step as you remember relative situations.

Step Two Tips

- The inventory is the most intensive part of this journey. Clear your schedule of unimportant or distracting things during this time. Allow life to slow down for a few weeks.
- **Do not begin your inventory during a major life event. This is not a good time to grow a family, get married, get a new job, go on a family vacation, or plan a move.**
- Set aside time each day to work until your inventory is complete.
- When making your lists, skip a line between each situation or person so you can add more information later.
- Be honest. Do not leave out an event, person, or situation because it is difficult. You are safe to express these things
- Give only enough information to trigger your recollection of the event, people, etc.
- It is okay to mention the same person on multiple lists or in several events.

Step Two Worksheet

Use the guide below to list the significant circumstances in your life. Bring any questions to your coach. Keep the descriptions of the events mentioned brief.

Inventory Lists: From your youngest memory to the present day

Part 1 – Create Six Lists
(You will reference these lists in parts 2 and 3 of this worksheet and in Step Three.)

1) List significant people, events, places, or ideas that had a positive impact in your life.

2) List people, situations, or ideas that you resent. (Resentment is unresolved fear or anger.)

3) List people, situations, or ideas that hurt you.

4) List situations, people, events, places, or ideas that caused you to fear.

5) List people in which sexual conduct has caused harm to yourself or others.

6) List people *you* have harmed. (Do not include the sexual harms mentioned above.)

Part 2 – Causes and Effects

- Return to List One. Describe the circumstances around the items listed and explain how they affected you positively.

- Return to List Two. Describe the circumstances around the items listed and why they angered you.

- Return to List Three. For each item listed, describe the type of harm you experienced and the cause of your hurt.

- Return to List Four. Describe the circumstances around the items listed and how they caused fear.

- Return to List Five. For each item listed, explain the nature of the sexual conduct and how it caused harm. Note: If you are the victim of rape or abuse, you are not at fault. Write about the harm caused *to* you.

- Return to List Six. Describe the circumstances around the items listed. In what way(s) were you responsible for causing the harm?

Part 3 – Messages

- Go back through *each list*. For each item describe the messages you received from the situation. How did this circumstance affect how you perceive your value and identity? How did it affect your character? How did the situation change your view of another person?

   ➢ **KEEP THESE LISTS! You will use them throughout this book!**

If you are confused by this step, ask your coach for a sample worksheet.

Lesson 22 — The Third Inventory Step

The Third Step

Completing this step of your inventory will be the most freeing thing you ever do. You will bring the darkness in your life into the light, discover the buried truth behind each secret, confess it all to someone you trust, and release it all to the Lord, removing its power. Light changes our perspective, allowing us to see our life through new eyes.

> *And I will lead the blind in a way that they do not know, in paths that they have not known*
> *I will guide them. I will turn the darkness before them into light, the rough places into level ground.*
> *These are the things I do, and I do not forsake them. (Isaiah 42:16)*

Instructions for the *Step Three* – Rebuilt *Inventory Worksheet*
(You will need your lists from Step Two to complete this step.)

- ➢ Complete an inventory worksheet for each item in List 2 (resentments) and discuss them with your coach. (Your coach has a resentment activity.)
- ➢ Complete an inventory worksheet **for each item in Lists 3, 4, and 5** and discuss them with your coach.
- ➢ After completing every worksheet, your coach will work with you to compare the messages received from all your negative situations with the positive impacts in List 1. You will look for messages with the greatest influence in your life. Which messages speak the loudest in your mind? Which speak truth? Is the truth louder than the lies you believe?
- ➢ Examine the harms you caused in List 6. Work with your coach to see how strongholds from past experiences and beliefs influenced your actions.
- ➢ Next, your coach will lead you in an activity to release your past to the Lord, empowering you to move forward. (Keep your lists for additional activities.)
- ➢ After confessing your lists to the Lord, **let them go! Do not take them back!** A balloon cannot fly away if you hold on to the string!

Step Three Tips

- ➢ Record your thoughts and feelings before, during, and after the event occurred. Search for triggers and patterns in your thoughts, feelings, or situations
- ➢ Write your answers to the questions on the second page of the Step Three worksheet in your journal, adding thorough details.
- ➢ Set aside time daily to work on your inventory. It is the most important part of your journey, so devote your time and effort to it.
- ➢ **You may** continue **to move forward in this book while working on this step.** The remaining lessons in this book can help you navigate difficult emotions and overcome stuck points.
- ➢ **Do not worry about how long the inventory takes.** This is **your** journey; it moves at your pace.
- ➢ Do not move on to the next book until your inventory is completed.
- ➢ **Keep all your lists!** They will be used for additional activities.

> THIS WAY→ Your coach has a vital role in this step. He or she will guide you through two life-changing activities. Prepare a full day for each activity.

Step Three — *Rebuilt* Inventory Worksheet

You may make copies of the worksheet or use it as a guide for writing in your journal.

What happened? Describe the circumstance/situation.

_____

_____

Was there an offense? (Did someone wrong me or offend me? Did I wrong or offend someone else?) What was the exact nature of the wrong?

_____

_____

Is the offense real or perceived? What was my part or responsibility in this situation?

_____

_____

Select what triggered your response to the situation. Do/Did you feel:

- ☐ Fearful/Anxious
- ☐ Like a failure
- ☐ Not good enough
- ☐ Unliked/Unloved
- ☐ Rejected or Insecure
- ☐ Vulnerable

- ☐ Angry
- ☐ Defiant/Controlling/Prideful
- ☐ Suspicious
- ☐ Jealous/Envious
- ☐ Bitter/Resentful
- ☐ Threatened (financially, physically, emotionally, etc.)

- ☐ Lonely/Neglected
- ☐ Guilty/Shameful
- ☐ Loss
- ☐ Self-pity (feeling sorry for yourself)

How did I respond to this situation?

_____

_____

_____

Were You:
- ☐ Tired/Exhausted
- ☐ Hungry
- ☐ Hurt emotionally
- ☐ Hurt physically

What harm came from (or could come from) my response to the situation?

_____

_____

_____

_____

Were* Your *Responses:
- ☐ Selfish/Self-seeking
- ☐ Dishonest
- ☐ Inconsiderate/Lacking Compassion
- ☐ Lacking Self-control/Self-discipline
- ☐ Controlling or Manipulating Others
- ☐ Prideful (Rejecting counsel/ prideful self-reliance)
- ☐ Ambitious for social/relational gain
- ☐ Ambitious for financial gain

How could I have responded differently?

_____

_____

_____

Can I correct the damage caused by my response? *If so, how?*

_____

_____

Answer the questions that correspond with the "Do you feel" boxes you checked.

(For example, if you checked the boxes for anger and insecurity, you would answer the questions under number 1 and number 2 below.)

1. **Angry, bitter, or resentful**
   a) What is the emotion behind the anger?
   b) What are you resentful or bitter about?
   c) What past circumstances have fed into this resentment?

2. **Fearful anxious, insecure, rejected, vulnerable, threatened, suspicious, jealous, envious**
   a) What are you afraid will happen?
   b) What situations in the past have taught you to fear this result?

3. **Self-pity, shameful, guilty, not enough, a failure, unliked, or unloved**
   a) What past experiences are making you feel this way?
   b) Are you being fair to yourself? Is this feeling reasonable or is it self-pity?

4. **Defiance, controlling, prideful**
   a) What were/are you trying to control?
   b) What happened in the past that made you feel a need to control in this circumstance?

5. **Lonely, loss, neglected**
   a) What is missing that causes you to feel this way?
   b) What losses in your past may have fed into this feeling?

_____

_____

_____

_____

_____

_____

To change our behaviors, we must change the way we think about things. When we identify where our patterns of emotion and behavior come from, we can separate the truth from the lies. In the future when we find ourselves in a similar situation, we can think about the truth we have learned and reject the thoughts and feelings that have held us captive.

What are the wrong messages—lies—you are believing in this circumstance?

_____

_____

What truth should you believe?

_____

_____

Chapter Six

Problematic Thinking & Stuck Points

FRUSTRATION IS A LOCK

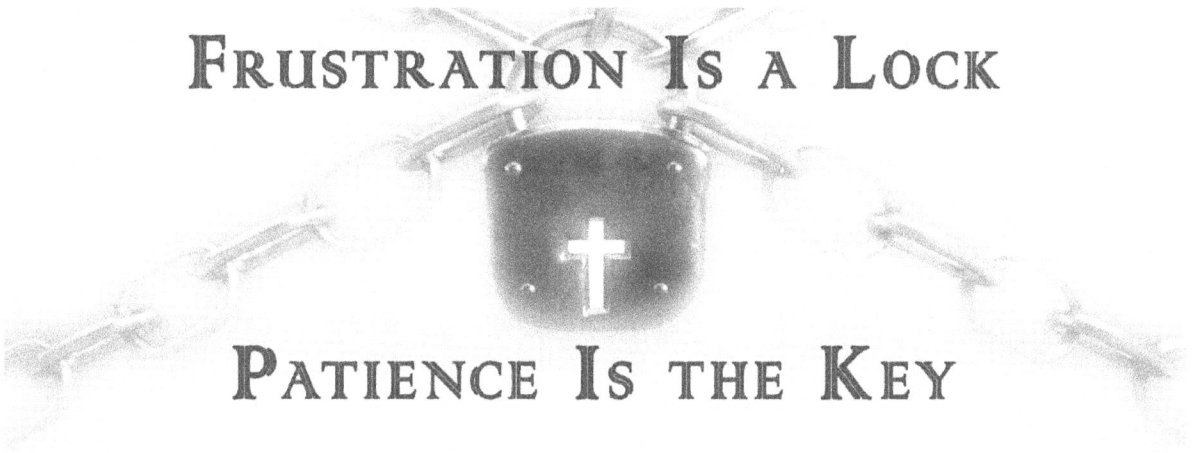

PATIENCE IS THE KEY

Not only that, but we rejoice in our sufferings, knowing that suffering produces endurance, and endurance produces character, and character produces hope, and hope does not put us to shame, because God's love has been poured into our hearts through the Holy Spirit who has been given to us. (Romans 5:3-5)

THE LORD IS THE LOCKSMITH, THE MAKER OF EVERY KEY

I am the vine; you are the branches. Whoever abides in me and I in him, he it is that bears much fruit, for apart from me you can do nothing. (John 15:5)

WHAT IS THIS FRUIT?

But the fruit of the Spirit is love, joy, peace, patience, kindness, goodness, faithfulness, gentleness, self-control; against such things there is no law. (Galatians 5:22-23)

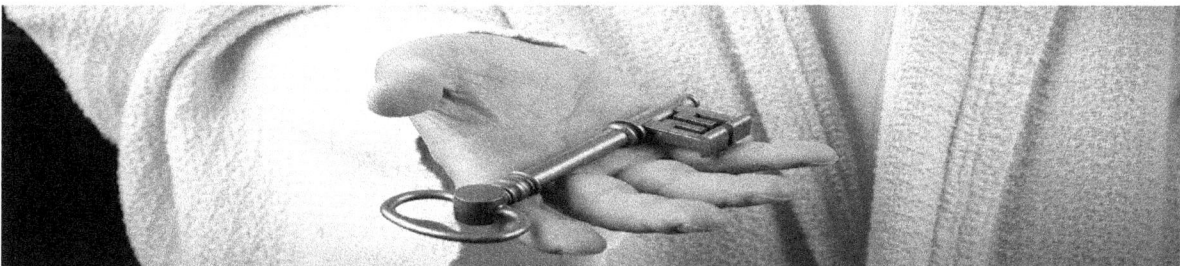

Lesson 23 — Problematic Thinking

Cognitive distortions are irrational, exaggerated patterns of thought that convince our mind to believe something untrue. These thought distortions go beyond simple negativity; **they may solidify a negative thought into a belief.**

There are many ways your thinking can distort your view of yourself, other people, and the world around you. Your ideas may have come from how you learned to relate in childhood, your life experiences, or when your belief system conflicts with the reality you experience. This is natural: Our mind attempts to make sense of what we do not understand and protect us from being hurt.

Some thoughts are automatic responses to an experience. These thoughts often line up with core beliefs about yourself, others, and the world. **Automatic thoughts are like a thinking habit.** You think without knowing you are thinking, and when these thoughts are negative, you may see even a positive event in a negative light. Thoughts that cause shame, bitterness, anger, fear, or insecurity may even lead to symptoms of depression or anxiety.

Check Your Thinking

➢ Read the "Problematic Thinking Patterns" worksheet.

➢ Check your inventory worksheets for thought patterns that may have caused misunderstandings or led to a toxic situation.

➢ This worksheet is not an exhaustive list but provides a good starting point to show the adverse effects that can result from your thinking.

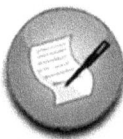

Use the "Problematic Thinking Worksheet" to examine ways you are thinking about your experiences this week.

1. **Watch for yourself or someone else to use one of these thinking patterns and write about it in your journal.**

2. **Look for an example of each type of distorted thinking.**

3. **On the worksheet, check the box next to the thought distortions you notice in yourself.**

Patterns of Problematic Thinking Worksheet

> **What thoughts are keeping you from a full recovery? These are your stuck points thoughts that keep you from forgiving another, or that keep you angry or insecure. Often, these thoughts originate from problematic thinking patterns.**

Directions:

Check the boxes next to a pattern you recognize in yourself and write an example for each checked pattern of how you have seen this pattern in your thinking.

☐ **Fortune-telling** – Jumping to conclusions, predicting or assuming a future outcome, or expecting the worst possible outcome to happen.
Clue words: "What if ..." statements.

☐ **Magnifying or Minimizing** – Magnifying is exaggerating a situation or blowing it out of proportion (i.e., making a mountain out of a molehill). Minimizing discounts the importance of something relevant. Often, they work together.
Example: Your team wins a game, but you minimize the win because you missed a goal, and you magnify your failure to get the goal.

☐ **Filtering** – Filtering out either positive or negative information about a situation.
Examples: The attitude that "having integrity won't pay my bills," or ignoring disciplinary action from a boss and only focusing on praise from a coworker (or vice-versa).

☐ **Polarized Thinking** – Oversimplifying things as good/bad, right/wrong. This is also referred to as "black and white" or "all or nothing" thinking. This way of thinking does not acknowledge gray areas or contributing circumstances.
Example: You accuse your spouse of failing to contribute to the family because they did not clean the house—ignoring the fact that your spouse was sick in bed most of the week.

☐ **Overgeneralization** – Drawing a conclusion based on one or two incidents. You perceive an incident as an event that will happen again and again, or as a pattern that will continue forever.
Clue words: "All," "None," "Always," "Never," "Every," "Constantly," "Can't," "Won't."
*Examples: "I **can't** get my bills right, **every** month I am late on something." Or someone cancels plans with you, and now you do not believe you can count on them.*

☐ **Personalization** – Taking what others do personally or comparing yourself with others. This thinking causes you to assume another's actions are a response to you or your behaviors. It may also be taking the blame for things outside of your responsibility or control.
Example: "She did not say anything at the meeting; I must have made her angry." "I should have been able to stop the accident."

- ☐ **Labeling** – When a person makes a mistake or something happens you dislike, you label the person, object, or situation based on that experience.
  Examples: *"The homework assignment is stupid." "She is so lazy." "I am a failure."*

- ☐ **Mind-reading** – Assuming the thoughts of others with no evidence of their opinions. This could be an assumption that a person has negative thoughts toward you, or assuming you know why a person acts a certain way.
  Examples: *"They will think I am worthless." "He must think I am stupid." "She has no good reason for staying home; she must be hiding something."*

- ☐ **Emotional Reasoning** – Considering your emotions as proof of the reality of a situation.
  Examples: *"I feel fear, so there is danger." "I feel stupid, so I am stupid."*

- ☐ ***Should* Statements** – Believing if you or someone else did something different, a situation would have had a better outcome. This thinking often places unrealistic expectations on yourself or others and may lead to shame, anger, or bitterness.
  Clue words: *"Should," "must," "ought."*
  Examples: *"I should have known that car was coming." "I should have known I couldn't trust him." "He ought to have more gratitude for everything I did for him."*

- ☐ **Blaming** – Holding other people responsible for your pain or seeing everything bad as someone else's fault entirely.
  Example: *"I tripped because you got in my way."*

- ☐ **Self-serving Bias** –Believing everything good that happens around you points to your excellent character, but negative events are out of your control.
- ☐ ***Example:*** *People with this thinking may refuse to admit their flaws and go to great lengths to prove they are not wrong. They may see themselves as always being right, believe their opinions are facts, or fail to consider the opinions or feelings of others*

- ☐ **Fallacy of Change** – The expectation that other people will change what they think or do to make you happy. This thinking insists on having its own way and may pressure or manipulate people to enforce it. Your happiness requires that another person change.
  Example: *Refusing to eat a meal with the family because you dislike the prepared food.*

- ☐ **Just World Fallacy** – The assumption that you get what you deserve in life, or that everything must be fair and equal. It is the belief that good things happen to good people, and bad things happen to bad people.
  Examples: *"They deserve to live in poverty because they do not work hard enough." "I went out on a date with my coworker because my husband cheated. It's only fair."*

Lesson 24 — Stuck Points

I Am Stuck and Cannot Get Past This! What Do I Do?

Why do we get stuck in unpleasant emotions and unhealthy behaviors? We become stuck because of the way we think. Our life experiences form our belief system. We filter everything that happens through that belief system. **Sometimes this filter makes it hard to see the truth.**

Most people have sought the approval of others to validate what they believe. We have a spiritual enemy who lies to us. We leave a door open to receive his lies when the opinions of a parent, spouse, friend, church leader, or anyone other than God shape our identity and worldviews. A person's opinion may seem right, but that does not mean it is truth.

> *There is a way that seems right to a man, but its end is the way to death.*
> *(Proverbs 14:12)*

Let us say, for example, that you have a natural talent and calling in a field. You apply for a job in that field and show proficient understanding of the job. The interviewer calls you back. You did not get the job, because you do not meet their experience requirements. Your mind forms a belief that you are unqualified for this career, and thus you give up seeking that kind of work.

In this situation, the enemy tells you the lie that you are unable—unqualified for this work. You hear the thought as your own and internalize it as a belief. The truth is that God gifted you for that career, and there are other jobs in the field for which you may qualify. However, the doubt and insecurity placed in your heart destroys your confidence. You no longer pursue what God created you to do. In this scenario, man's rejection opened a door for the enemy to frame your thinking in a detrimental way. Your belief that you are not good enough causes you to abandon your calling.

> *For am I now seeking the approval of man, or of God? Or am I trying to please man? If I were still trying to please man, I would not be a servant of Christ.*
> *(Galatians 1:10)*

> *Because there is no truth in him [the devil]. When he lies, he speaks out of his own character, for he is a liar and the father of lies.*
> *(John 8:44)*

> *And no wonder, for even Satan disguises himself as an angel of light.*
> *(2 Corinthians 11:14)*

> *But I am afraid that as the serpent deceived Eve by his cunning, your thoughts will be led astray from a sincere and pure devotion to Christ.*
> *(2 Corinthians 11:3)*

To get unstuck, you must:

> ➢ Recognize what you are thinking and believing
>
> ➢ See how those beliefs affect your emotional state and your actions
>
> ➢ Challenge those thoughts to recognize any lies you believe
>
> ➢ Submit the lies to God's truth and **choose to** believe the Lord's report
>
> ➢ Change your self-talk with truth (not just positive words)

The goal is to change what you say to yourself, choose to believe truth, and form different thoughts about your experiences and how you make sense of those experiences. Many times, you may not be aware of your self-talk or what you are thinking or believing. This chapter will help you **identify and challenge your thoughts**.

If evil looked like evil, you would flee from it.
If a lie looked like a lie, you would never believe it.

As you go through your inventory, you may find things that are interfering with your recovery or keeping you stuck. These are your "stuck points." Often your stuck points contribute to the "things you want to change" list from your heart check.

Create a page in your journal to use as a "Stuck Points" log.
You will add to this list as you work on your inventory and
pull from this list as you tackle your problematic thinking.

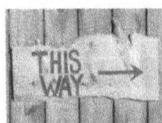

Stuck points may be conflicts between your beliefs before and after a traumatic experience. If you have experienced trauma that is keeping you stuck, tell your coach. Your coach will have additional resources to help you.

Discover and Overcome Stuck Points
First, Know What You Think

How Thought, Emotion, and Behavior Relate
Say the following situation occurs: Someone asks you to speak at an event in front of about 100 people. The situation triggers the thought, "I am going to mess this up." That thought leads to an emotion, and you experience nervousness. You then decline the opportunity to speak. The thought led to your emotion, which influenced the choice you made not to speak.

However, sometimes an emotion occurs without a thought to evoke the emotion. It may even seem unrelated to the current situation. Not all our thoughts are **conscious thoughts**, where we hear the words in our head. Beliefs stored in our **subconscious mind** may also trigger emotions. **Beliefs**, whether they are true or not true, are solid ideas that influence the way we see things for as long as we hold that belief. In the previous example, you may not think the words, "I am going to mess this up." But you may see yourself as a failure, and if so, this belief will make you nervous when speaking before a large group.

Discover Your Thoughts

To discover the thoughts behind the emotion, ask yourself why you have this emotion. What are you saying to yourself that causes these feelings? Is it the current situation or something outside of the situation that causes your mind to process this way?

To discover our thoughts and challenge and replace problematic thinking, we will use the "K.C.R." worksheets on the following pages.

Worksheet K – Know Your Thoughts

Use this worksheet to figure out what you are thinking or feeling in any given situation.

- If you are more aware of your feelings, fill in that column first. Then trace back the situation and discover the message you were saying to yourself.

- Use this worksheet as soon as you recognize a problem, so you are more likely to remember what you were saying to yourself. You may have more than one thought or emotion for a situation.

- Emotions are usually one-word answers. For example, "I feel sad" represents an emotion. "I feel like I can never do anything right." Is a thought or belief it is not an emotion.

A Situation *Something Happens*	B Thought/Belief *What I tell myself*	C Emotion *What I feel*

**Do not try to analyze if the thought is right or wrong;
simply identify what you are thinking.**

(Ask your coach for samples of completed worksheets and discuss your answers with your coach)

Worksheet C – Challenge Your thoughts

Now that you have identified what you think, challenge those thoughts. Are they the truth?
Answer all *relevant* questions below for each belief listed in column B on your "K" worksheet.

Situation *(Column A)*: _____

1. What was your part in this?

2. What part did other's play in the situation?

3. What are the facts of the situation? What new information, if any, has come to light?

Belief: _____ How much do you believe this thought? _____%

4. What other past experiences led to or supported this belief?

5. Does this belief fall into a problematic thinking pattern? _____ Explain.

6. Is your belief a habitual response, based in feelings, or based in facts?

7. What evidence supports this belief?   Is your source of information reliable?

8. What evidence suggests this belief is not true?

9. What assumptions were made?

10. Are you using words that are extreme/exaggerated (always, never, should, must, etc.)?

11. Are you taking a situation out of context, (focusing only on one aspect/irrelevant factors)?

12. Realistically, what are the chances your concerns will happen?

13. Are your interpretations accurate, or could you have misinterpreted the facts?

14. What does the bible say about you or the situation? Does it line up with your belief?

15. If your child, friend, or loved one came to you with your belief, what would you tell them?

Worksheet R – Replace Your Thoughts

After examining the situations and your beliefs in worksheet "C", you may begin to see some lies that you have believed. It is important to take everything you believe and hold it up to God's word. Does it line up with what the scripture says?

For instance:

❖ If shame is part of your beliefs, does it belong to you? Are you guilty? Blame goes to those with **responsibility and intent**. If something bad happened and you have some responsibility in it, yet you did not intend for it to happen, you should not carry guilt.

> *"Then Jesus said, 'Father, forgive them, for they do not know what they are doing.'" (Luke 23:34)*

> *"For the LORD sees not as man sees: man looks on the outward appearance, but <u>the LORD looks on the heart</u>." (1 Samuel 16:7)*

❖ If you are guilty of something, do you believe the lie that you are too bad for forgiveness? Do you believe that your mistakes define who you are? In Christ, when you take responsibility for your wrongs and repent *(turn away from it)* the Lord is faithful and just to forgive you. If you have remorse and turn away from wrongdoing, you no longer need to carry the weight of guilt.

> *"If we confess our sins, he is faithful and just to forgive us our sins and to cleanse us from all unrighteousness." (1 John 1:9)*

> *"For godly grief produces a repentance that leads to salvation without regret, whereas worldly grief produces death." (2 Corinthians 7:10)*

Consider the situation you wrote in the A column on your "K" worksheet.

- What is your true responsibility for the situation?

- What was the actual responsibility of others involved?

- Whom do you need to forgive? Do you need to forgive yourself?

- Do you need to seek forgiveness from the Lord, or make amends for past wrongs?

- What lies are you believing?

- How can you think differently about the situation?

- What is the truth? What can you say instead of the original thought/belief (from column B)?

- How strongly do you believe this new thought? _____%
- How much do you now believe the original thought? _____%
- Choose and memorize a verse that speaks about your problem or helps solidify the truth/new belief.

Chapter Seven

Self-control

Lesson 25 — Overwhelming Emotion

Sometimes life happens too quickly, emotions are too strong, anger is too overwhelming, or the fear is too great, for us to analyze a situation. When a moment of life becomes this overpowering, it is difficult to function or even pray.

Anger and fear are two damaging emotions when they are misunderstood, and they can keep us trapped in a deep web of false beliefs, sometimes leading us to fear or blame God. These emotions can drive us to a place where we cannot pray and seek the Lord, giving the enemy free rein. Then he can speak any lie he wants into our ears. One thought feeds another, until the situation seems utterly hopeless. Have you ever been there?

This chapter will introduce different biblical strategies for self-control—strategies that can stop your mind from spinning before you lose control. These are "in the moment" tools. If you learned other **healthy strategies** for handling emotions that work for you, continue to use them. However, many times our coping mechanisms **are not healthy**. Consider the impact of your coping skills.

Questions to Ponder

25.1) How often do you lose control of your thoughts or actions when experiencing anger?

25.2) How often do you lose control of your thoughts or actions when experiencing fear or an unknown situation?

25.3) Write about a recent situation in which you felt your emotions spin you out of control.

25.4) Thinking back, can you identify what first triggered the emotion (what started it)?

Self-control is a fruit of the Spirit. The ability to control yourself is only possible with the Lord. Your heart can change, but you cannot change it. In our flesh we can control behavior temporarily, but only the Spirit of God can change the corruption in our heart that drives our behavior. We cannot change our sin nature any more than a leopard can change his spots.

For I do not understand my own actions. For I do not do what I want, but I do the very thing I hate. (Romans 7:15)

Can the Ethiopian change his skin, or the leopard his spots? Neither are you able to do good—you who are accustomed to doing evil. (Jeremiah 13:23, BSB)

Questions to Ponder

25.5) What are some healthy ways you cope with difficult emotions?

25.6) What are some detrimental ways you cope with difficult emotions?

25.7) How have poor coping skills harmed you and those around you?

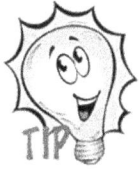

> ## Self-control is freedom.
>
> Emotions can become your prison.
> Self-control is freedom *not* to respond instead of giving your emotions control.
>
> > It is freedom **NOT** to act in anger.
> >
> > It is freedom **NOT** to stay home out of fear.
> >
> > It is **NOT** legalism; it is **NOT** a prison.

Emotions: Are They Good or Bad?

God created us in His image, and He has emotions. He gets angry, He loves, and He grieves. Jesus wept at the death of Lazarus and turned over tables in the temple when there was injustice in His Father's house. It is not a sin to have emotions; it is sin if we act on those emotions in a wrong way.

> *For we do not have a high priest who is unable to sympathize with our weaknesses, but*
> *one who in every respect has been tempted as we are, yet without sin.*
> *(Hebrews 4:15)*

Many people find emotional regulation extremely difficult. Even the most emotionally stable people have moments where emotions dictate their actions. Unlike us, God deals well with His emotions. He is always just and good regardless of His feelings.

> *The anger of man does not produce the and kill and righteousness of God.*
> *(Ephesians 4:26)*

Emotions are beneficial in that they give us information. Anger alerts us to injustice; fear alerts us to danger; grief and pain teach compassion; love teaches us about the Lord.

In our sin nature, we misuse our emotions. Fear may compel us to control and use people, to manipulate circumstances, or to protect ourselves from perceived dangers aroused by our jealousy or insecurity. Pride and selfishness may stir anger when we do not like the circumstance or how people behave or respond. Anger leads to hate, gossip, slander, and other forms of sin.

We have an enemy whispering in our ears. His main tactic for destruction involves our thoughts and emotions. He feeds on our fears and insecurities, telling lies that make a normal situation seem like something it is not. Jesus came to overcome the enemy and the power of sin and death in us. The enemy tries to use our emotions against us, **hoping we will reject the abundant life Christ wants us to possess**. When we understand our emotions, **they can alert us to and stop the plans of the enemy**. The more we understand why we feel as we do, the more we can spot deception and false thinking.

> *The thief comes only to steal destroy. I came that they may have life*
> *and have it abundantly. (John 10:10)*

91

Emotional Control

Do not allow your emotions to draw you into sin, fear, or anger. Do not allow them to continue unabated without understanding or resolution. Recognize and accept your emotions. If you fear or reject your feelings, you may bury them. Suppressed emotion causes anxiety and other mental health issues. It is important to acknowledge emotion, **but if you do not control the emotion, it will control you**.

Be angry and do not sin; do not let the sun go down on your anger.
(James 1:20)

For God gave us a spirit not of fear but of power and love and self-control.
(2 Timothy 1:7)

Questions to Ponder

25.8) Question your feelings. What is the most prevalent emotion you experience?

25.9) Do you shut down emotion?

25.10) Do your emotional responses come long after the situation?

25.11) Are you an emotional person? Do your emotions control your decision-making process?

How Behavior Works

To break the chains of codependency, anger, mental illness, addiction, and so on, we must **literally break a chain**. A situation, circumstance, or physical sensation triggers a **thought**, and that thought triggers a **feeling/emotion**, which triggers a **behavior/action**, which triggers a **consequence**. The consequence often triggers another thought, which triggers another emotion, which triggers another behavior and another consequence. The cycle continues, tightening our emotional shackles and leading us into a deep, tangled web of confusion.

Detrimental thoughts are the start of that chain. It is best to take those thoughts captive at the chain's beginning. The more you allow thoughts to go unchecked, the longer your chain and the more links you must destroy to release yourself from your chain. The book of James illustrates this process:

But each person is tempted [thoughts] when he is lured and enticed by his own
desire [emotions]. Then desire when it has conceived gives birth to sin [behavior]
and sin when it is fully grown brings forth death [consequence].
(James 1: 14 – 15)

Question to Ponder

25.12) Write about a time when you experienced this process play out in your own life.

Trust and Humility

The best weapon against overwhelming emotions is to humble yourself and trust in the Lord. Do not assume you know the answers or that the world has your answers. You may have part of it right, and the world may have part of it right. God, who created everything, is the only one with the big picture and all the answers. God cares for you. Leaning on His truth will bring you peace and healing.

Trust in the LORD with all your heart, and do not lean on your own understanding. In all your ways acknowledge him, and he will make straight your paths. Be not wise in your own eyes; fear the LORD, and turn away from evil. It will be healing to your flesh and refreshment to your bones. (Proverbs 3:5 – 8)

Blessed be the God and Father of our Lord Jesus Christ, the Father of mercies and God of all comfort, who comforts us in all our affliction, so that we may be able to comfort those who are in any affliction, with the comfort with which we ourselves are comforted by God. For as we share abundantly in Christ's sufferings, so through Christ we share abundantly in comfort too. (2 Corinthians 1:3 – 5)

Questions to Ponder

25.13) Do you believe God cares about you and cares for you?

25.14) What are some ways that the Lord has taken care of you in the past?

Lesson 26 — Coping Strategies

How Should We Deal with Emotion?

Scripture shows us the correct way to deal with emotions in first Peter:

> *Humble yourselves, therefore, under the mighty hand of God so that at the proper time he may exalt you, casting all your anxieties on him, because he cares for you. Be sober-minded; be watchful. Your adversary the devil prowls around like a roaring lion, seeking someone to devour. Resist him, firm in your faith, knowing that the same kinds of suffering are being experienced by your brotherhood throughout the world. And after you have suffered a little while, the God of all grace, who has called you to his eternal glory in Christ, will himself restore, confirm, strengthen, and establish you.*
> *(1 Peter 5:6 – 10)*

Let emotions alert you to a situation and give you information:

➢ **Humble yourself**. Do not rely on your way of thinking to understand. Seek God's wisdom and give your concerns about the situation to Him. Tell Him how you feel! He cares for you, and He will help you.

➢ **Keep your mind sober.** Do not use alcohol or drugs to run away from your emotions. *(Note: This is referring to self-medicating. Never stop taking medications prescribed under a qualified physician's care without your doctor's guidance. This may cause serious harm.)*

   o A sober mind is also a steady, sound mind. Do not allow your thoughts to spin out of control. Take them to the Lord first.

➢ **Keep guard against the lies of the enemy.** He will try to spin you up or use your emotions against you. Do not let him.

➢ **Resist the enemy:**

   o Trust that the Lord will keep you in whatever you are going through.

   o Know you are not alone in your pain; God is with you, and others have suffered what you are suffering and come through it.

   o Understand that your suffering is only for a short time. When the season is over, God Himself will restore, confirm, strengthen, and establish you.

   o Seek and believe truth.

The following strategies are the first steps in managing your emotions.
The moment you feel negative emotions or face temptation,
S.T.O.P. then **T.H.I.N.K.**

Questions to Ponder

Read the following two strategies, (STOP and THINK) and put them into practice.

26.1) Write about using the strategies.

26.2) How did the strategies help you?

26.3) Where did you find the strategies difficult to implement?

To remember the ways in which the Lord has blessed you, cared for you, and comforted you, is like a memorial to God commemorating all He has done in your life.

Create/Use a praise journal.

Every day, write the ways you can give thanks to the Lord in your journal!

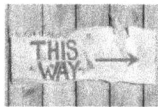

Share your Praise Journal with your coach.
Read your journal when you have times of doubt.

Strategy: S.T.O.P.

*The acrostic S.T.O.P. can help you remember what to do when a strong emotion comes as a surprise. It is important **to stop at the initial thought** before the emotions are get too powerful and spin you out of control.*

Treat your emotions like a stop sign. You are not trying to stop the emotion; you are stopping your thinking. When an emotion surprises you or appears negative, recognize it as you would a stop sign when you are driving. The vehicle of thought must come to a complete stop! When thoughts spin up, it is exceedingly difficult to regain control.

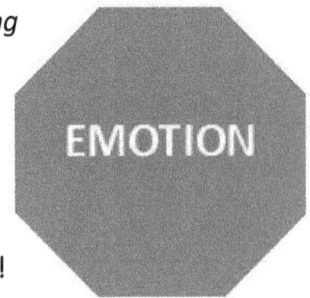

Stay

Stay at the feet of Jesus. Become grounded in the present. Do not hang out in the past or look toward future concerns. Focus on the here and now. Find a point of focus, like the chair you are sitting on, for example. The only thing required of you is simply to breathe. Put your concerns on a shelf in your mind. Wait until you are in a better place or the Lord directs you to act before taking the concern off your shelf.

> *They who wait for the LORD shall renew their strength; they shall mount up with wings like eagles; they shall run and not be weary; they shall walk and not faint. (Isaiah 40:31)*

Trust

Trust that God has it. This is the power of letting. **Let** God hear your emotion, **let** Him know your concern, your anger, or your fear, and **let** Him take responsibility for the outcome. In things out of your control, do not search for ways to force the situation into your control. Remember, the Lord knows what is best, and He sees the situation clearer than you do.

> *Trust in the LORD with all your heart, and do not lean on your own understanding.*
> *In all your ways acknowledge him, and he will make straight your paths. (Proverbs 3:5 – 6)*

Observe

Observe the conditions that could contribute to the emotion. Are you tired? Hungry? Sick? Overwhelmed? Did you take medicine? Ladies, are you near your cycle? All these things can magnify the emotion you feel. Examine the situation. What is happening that you dislike? What is concerning you? Is the emotion you are experiencing out of proportion to the circumstance?

> *But if we judged ourselves truly, we would not be judged. (2 Corinthians 11:31)*

Pray

Pray that the Lord will reveal what you need to know or the actions you should take. Be humble and do not lean on your own understanding. Remain calm: Time is on your side. Wait for an answer from the Lord.

> *If any of you lacks wisdom, let him ask God, who gives generously to all without reproach, and it will be given him. (James 1:5)*

Strategy: T.H.I.N.K.
First use the STOP strategy, then you can THINK.

Turn

Turn the emotion into information. What information does the emotion tell you? What are your actual beliefs about yourself or your situation? Seek the Lord for the truth about the situation.

> *But I say, walk by the Spirit, and you will not gratify the desires of the flesh. (Galatians 5:16)*

Honest

Be honest and humble. What are you learning about yourself from the emotion? Are you being inconsiderate or self-centered? Are you insecure or worried? Are your expectations reasonable?

> *If we say we have no sin, we deceive ourselves, and the truth is not in us. (1 John 1:8)*

Investigate

Investigate all the options. Identify your assumptions and look for alternative plausible explanations. What information is still unknown? Are the expectations of others reasonable? How could the enemy be using your emotion to cause harm? What lies are you hearing or trusting?

> *The simple believes everything, but the prudent gives thought to his steps. (Proverbs 14:15)*

No

No snap decisions. Learn to tell yourself no. Step back and take time to assess the situation. Gather your thoughts, ask questions, and get truthful information. Powerful emotions tempt us to jump to conclusions. You cannot take back a snap response, and it often will do more damage than good. Before you act, give yourself a cooling-off period to process your emotions and what happened to trigger them. Allow God time to move on your behalf in the situation. Avoiding impulsiveness prevents choices we regret. **The path of least regret is rarely the easy or quick path.**

> *If one gives an answer before he hears, it is his folly and shame. (Proverbs 18:13)*

Keep

Keep sober-minded to prepare your mind for action. Guard your mind by focusing your thoughts on the Kingdom of God and whatever is true, honorable, just, pure, lovely, commendable, excellent, and anything worthy of praise (see Philippians 4:8).

> *Therefore, preparing your minds for action, and being sober-minded, set your hope fully on the grace that will be brought to you at the revelation of Jesus Christ. (1 Peter 1:13)*

Chapter Eight

Perseverance

Lesson 27 — Persevere

What is perseverance? The Scripture uses words like "steadfastness," "endurance," and "patience." The Merriam-Webster dictionary says perseverance is persistence in doing something despite difficulty or delay in achieving success. It is hard to keep doing the right things, to keep having faith, when the answers seem far away. It is hard to keep on when the battle seems endless, and to keep standing up in our weakness. Yet we prosper if we do not give up.

And let us not grow weary of doing good, for in due season we will reap,
if we do not give up. (Galatians 6:9)

We Must Persevere

The Lord allows us to experience trials to test us and strengthen our character. We enter the Kingdom of God through many tribulations. (Tribulation: A cause or state of great trouble or suffering.)

In the world you will have tribulation. But take heart; I have overcome the world.
(John 16:33)

When you do something new, prepare a new product, or promote a new program, you test it, right? You will run trials to check what works and remove any bugs. Tests and trials are also a necessary part of the process of transformation to make us a new creation in Christ.

Perseverance through Difficulty Is the Growing Pains of Character

The Lord knows the hidden things in our heart that we struggle to see. We may think we have overcome a character defect, but when the right trial comes along, that defect can rise to the surface again. Our trials and stresses shed light on our weaknesses, helping us to see where we are and how much we have grown. Each trial we face brings us deeper into the root of our character defects so God can do a complete work in our hearts.

The Lord does not allow trials and tests so He can grade our progress. Our trials benefit us, helping us see where we need to grow and how far we have come, refining us, making us perfect and complete. They strengthen our faith, nurture our love, make our hope certain, and mold us into a reflection of Jesus—the person God predestined us to become to receive His eternal promise.

More than that, we rejoice in our sufferings, knowing that suffering produces endurance, and endurance produces character, and character produces hope, and hope does not put us to shame, because God's love has been poured into our hearts through the Holy Spirit who has been given to us. (Romans 5:3 – 5)

For you know that the testing of your faith produces steadfastness. And let steadfastness have its full effect, that you may be perfect and complete, lacking in nothing. (James 1:3 – 4)

For those whom he foreknew he also predestined <u>to be conformed to the image of his Son</u>, in order that he might be the firstborn among many brothers. (Romans 8:29)

When we persevere, we are blessed with eternal victory!

And you will be hated by all for my name's sake.
But the one who endures to the end will be saved. (Matthew 10:22)

Be the Tree!

Blessed is the man who <u>trusts in the LORD</u>, whose <u>trust is the LORD</u>. He is like a tree
planted by water, that sends out its roots by the stream, and does not fear when heat
comes, for its leaves remain green, and is not anxious in the year of drought, for it does
not cease to bear fruit. (Jeremiah 17:7 – 8)

He is like a tree planted by streams of water that yields its fruit in its season, and
its leaf does not wither. In all that he does, he prospers. (Psalm 1:1 – 3)

Perseverance starts with trust. God is the only place worthy of your trust. We trust in Him, but **He IS also our trust**. If you have a dozen eggs, you can put some eggs in a basket and others in your refrigerator, in a pan, on your counter, and even save a couple to throw at someone's house. It is the same with trust. You can put trust in the Lord and put trust in your shelter, in weapons, in your skill, in your wisdom, in your family, or in your friends. Jeremiah is telling us to trust in the Lord, but also to make the Lord the place which holds all our trust. Our trust **is** the Lord, **like putting all your eggs in one basket; you put all you have in Him.**

Scripture compares perseverance to a tree planted by water. The tree planted can stand in the heat; it does not wither from drought; instead, it always produces fruit. The tree's roots keep it connected to the source of life-giving water. **The Lord is our source of life.** When we stay connected to our source, we can stand the heat of the refiner's fire and will not wither in times of lack. Our lives will never stop bearing fruit. We will prosper in all we do because we stay grounded in our source.

And he is before all things, and in him all things hold together. (Colossians 1:17)

Stay Grounded in Your Source

You cast off many things during your inventory, emptying yourself of past pain, lies, fear, sin, and guilt. Now it is time to put on something new. You must replace what you took off, filling the holes left in your heart. The trick is to fill them with suitable things.

First, you put off your old self and renewed your mind in truth. This was your inventory and heart check. It is plausible that you will discover more things to put off as you walk through life with God. The process of removing lies and renewing your mind is ongoing. After putting off your old self, you must put on your new self in Christ. The book of Romans tells us the **first thing** you put on is Jesus, so you can be transformed into His likeness.

To put off your old self, which belongs to your former manner of life and is corrupt through deceitful desires, and to be renewed in the spirit of your minds, and to put on the new self, created after the likeness of God in true righteousness and holiness. (Ephesians 4:22 – 24)

But put on the Lord Jesus Christ, and make no provision for the flesh, to gratify its desires.
(Romans 13:14)

Jesus is our source. Once we put Him on, we stand strong by putting on the whole armor of God. **This is how we become the tree planted by the water**.

Put on the whole armor of God, that you may be able to stand
against the schemes of the devil. (Ephesians 6:11)

Read Ephesians 6:11 - 18

This armor, mentioned in Ephesians, is our relationship with God. The **belt of truth** keeps the armor on. Rebuking the enemy's lies in exchange for God's truth, knowing His word, and living a life of honesty and integrity, keeps the other pieces of armor in place. The **breastplate of righteousness** protects your heart, keeping your heart in check so no sin can creep in and take hold. Your **shoes** guard your walk. Walk in the footsteps of Jesus in every moment of your day. The **gospel of peace** keeps you confident. In every circumstance, keep your **shield of faith**—your trust in God. Every dart the enemy can throw will bounce off this shield. Guard your mind with the **helmet of salvation**. The enemy attacks your mind, the place which births emotion, desire, sin, doubt, love, and hate. When you think wrongly, the enemy gains a foothold, and everything goes wrong. Rest assured, you are the Lord's, and His Word is true for you.

Your offensive tool is the **sword of the Spirit**, fighting against enemy's attacks. The Holy Spirit deciphers God's Word, speaking directly into your life. Finally, **cover everything in prayer** and pray for your brothers and sisters in Christ.

When you dress in God's armor, you can stand!

<u>Questions to Ponder</u>
Read the following CHOICE strategy and put it into practice.

27.1) Write about using the strategy.

27.2) How did the strategy help you?

27.3) Where did you find the strategy difficult to implement?

Strategy: C.H.O.I.C.E.

You will stand strong with the Lord each day when you choose well. **Choose** Him first in each moment, and you will persevere every day, in everything.

Character

Choose excellent character in trial. STOP and THINK so you do not react in your flesh, but in the wisdom and love of the Lord.

> *But the one who looks into the perfect law, the law of liberty, and perseveres, being no hearer who forgets but a doer who acts, he will be blessed in his doing. (James 1:25)*

Hope

Place your hope in the Lord. Remember the promises of God and count on them.

> *Rejoice in hope, be patient in tribulation, be constant in prayer. (Romans 12:12)*

Optimism

Optimism in trials brings us joy, because we are confident that the Lord will work through everything for our benefit. Keep a heart of gratitude, remembering the Lord's provisions. Know with certainty that He finishes the work He starts. Optimism comes from hope. Hope deferred makes the heart sick.

> *Count it all joy, my brothers, when you meet trials of various kinds, for you know that the testing of your faith produces steadfastness. And let steadfastness have its full effect, that you may be perfect and complete, lacking in nothing. (James 1:2 – 4)*

Immovable

Be the immovable tree. Stand firm and do not allow your faith to waiver. The Lord has your back. He is the strength and the source allowing you to stand.

> *Therefore, my beloved brothers, be steadfast, immovable, always abounding in the work of the Lord, knowing that in the Lord your labor is not in vain. (1 Corinthians 15:58)*

Connected

Stay connected to your source. Keep the Word of the Lord in you and live your life in Him. Allow everything you do and all that you are to come from Him.

> *If you abide in me, and my words abide in you, ask whatever you wish, and it will be done for you. (John 15:7)*

Escape

Escape from flesh temptations. The Lord provides a way to escape temptation, including temptations to doubt God, fear circumstances, act in anger, or gratify a desire contrary to the Lord.

> *No temptation has overtaken you that is not common to man. God is faithful, and he will not let you be tempted beyond your ability, but with the temptation he will also provide the way of escape, that you may be able to endure it. (1 Corinthians 10:13)*

Chapter Nine

Anger Management

Lesson 28 — Dealing with Anger

Why Do We Get Angry?

Many circumstances trigger anger. Anger may **result from an injustice** perpetrated against us or another we love. **Or it can be motivated by a desire not to feel guilt or shame.** To **avoid looking** at our own sins, mistakes, or flaws, we may shift the blame to other people or circumstances, projecting our anger onto the victim of our wrongs.

Anger is a way our mind protects us from feeling another emotion, such as fear or pain. The adrenaline rush that comes with anger covers up disturbing feelings and **provides a sense of invulnerability**, which allows us to escape upsetting emotions in the moment. This anger is a **secondary emotion**, and to deal with it, we must first expose the emotion that triggered it.

Remember the acrostic **H.U.F.F.** to discover what is hiding beneath your anger:

- **H**urt – Physical or emotional pain, accusations, guilt, shame, feeling disregarded, unimportant, devalued, rejected, or unlovable.

- **U**nfairness – Unfair circumstances, not getting your way, envy (someone else has what you want), or believing nothing is fair in life.

- **F**ear – Feeling powerless, anxious, worried, intimidated, jealous, fearful of loss or the future, or other frightening circumstances.

- **F**rustration – Consistent mistakes, failure, circumstances not working out the way you want, hopelessness, disappointment, helplessness, feeling out of control, feeling life is too difficult, or experiencing many minor irritations and daily hassles.

In anger, when a person offends or hurts you, you may retaliate by returning the same hurt. For example, if a person belittles or rejects you, you may find something for which to ridicule or reject them. You are no longer the one demeaned; they are. A person who feels powerless or insecure may act out in a fit of rage to feel empowered and safe. Anger responses push your burden onto another while giving you a false sense of control. Your burden still exists beneath the mask of rage, but now it has become another's burden as well.

Anger begets more anger. Those receiving your anger often retaliate in anger. They feel threatened, responding with their own defensive actions, and escalating the conflict. Sometimes, however, people may flee your wrath, responding with hurt and fear instead of lashing out. They may distance themselves from you to escape your anger.

Defining Anger and Aggression

Anger can range from mild irritation to fierce rage and may lead to aggression. It is important to catch your anger right away before it escalates. **Aggression is deliberate harm to another**, physical or otherwise. Common aggressive behaviors include violence, breaking things, yelling, and screaming, but aggression may also appear passive.

Passive aggression is manipulation, which manifests as seeking revenge, sarcasm, ridicule, shunning, or slander. People often display passive aggressive behaviors with bitterness and resentment. They may respond by refusing, delaying, or being inefficient in doing something with the intent to cause another harm or "get them back." An example of passive aggressive behavior is refusing to do a task until the one who benefits from the task does something you want first. Passive aggressive people do not discuss their concerns. They may rationalize their behavior as "fairness" or deny their anger altogether.

Righteous Anger

We may become angry when people hurt us through no fault of our own, or when we see an injustice that goes unpunished. People disrespect the God we love, the innocent get hurt , and evil prevails. What angers the Lord can and should anger us. While we may justify this anger, when we respond to it with bitterness, resentment, and hate, we are sinning in our anger. To react in anger makes a situation worse, preventing others from understanding our feelings or resolving the issue. Whether it is selfish or righteous, we must not sin in our anger.

> *Be angry and do not sin; do not let the sun go down on your anger,*
> *and give no opportunity to the devil. (Ephesians 4:26 – 27)*

It may seem like ignoring or avoiding anger keeps peace. The reality is that avoiding a problem allows anger to fester inside. As you stew on the situation, you give the enemy the opportunity to plant thoughts and schemes, amplifying the conflict in your mind and tempting you to act in a way that escalates the situation. Not letting the sun go down on your anger means you should deal with your feelings right away. This prevents escalation or avoidance, which aggravates the situation. The longer you hold on to anger, the more opportunity you give the devil to manipulate it.

Anger Misconceptions

One common misconception about anger is that people believe they just need to vent, and everything will be better. It is not good to suppress or ignore your anger, but it is just as harmful to vent your anger or unleash your rage on another. Not only do you crush another's spirit, but **every time you lash out, it reinforces your aggressive behavior**. You form a belief that you must act out or the anger will consume you. When we frequently reinforce detrimental anger responses, they become automatic. Anger becomes our "go-to" for dealing with any situation we dislike. **Anger becomes a habit.**

Anger is not hereditary, but witnessing extreme anger responses as a child can cause it to become a habitual response for you. You may be unaware of the force behind the anger driving your behavior. If this is true of you, attempt to realize the moment you feel hostility and take your anger captive. Healthy handling of anger prevents it from festering like a neglected wound, releasing the anger in a way that resolves the problem.

False Invulnerability

Another misconception about anger is believing your intimidation and aggression make people respect you or treat you well. You may feel that being enraged makes people listen or give you what you want or need. The truth is that, while angry reactions may cause people to fear you, pretend to like you, or guard their words around you, **they do not respect you for your anger**. Almost everyone responds better when treated kindly. Even if a person is compliant, angry bullying breeds resentment.

Uncontrollable Anger

It is a lie that you cannot help how you respond or control yourself when angry. Anger is not destructive behavior, nor does it cause aggression. The intensity of the emotion makes it seem beyond your ability to control, but anger is like any other emotion. Despite how it feels, anger is only a signal giving you information that alerts you to a problem. You can **choose to control** how you express anger and handle it in a way that does not cause physical or emotional abuse.

> Verbal or physical aggression, damaging property, or hurting people is not anger. These are behaviors resulting from anger when we do not manage the emotion in a healthy, biblical way.

You must separate anger from behaviors, recognizing that they are distinct from one another. You cannot prevent anger, but **you can choose and control how you respond to that anger.** This realization empowers you to stop your anger from escalating or festering.

> ➢ **Recognize** anger at the first sign of wrong thinking, before it overwhelms you.
> ➢ **Choose** to deal with the emotions behind the anger.
> ➢ **Choose** to resolve issues instead of allowing anger to fester.

Deal with Your Anger

If you struggle with anger or it seems out of control, pay close attention to what triggered the anger. When did you first feel irritation? Are you responding without thinking or out of habit? Is your feeling based on wrong thinking or truth? What is the emotion or stronghold (the influencing belief) behind the anger? What triggered your anger? Is your anger justified? How can you resolve this situation?

How Angry Are You?

Consider your anger like a ladder with ten rungs. The ground represents complete calm with no irritation or resentment. At the first sign of irritation or annoyance, you climbed to the bottom rung of your ladder. The top rung of the ladder represents explosive anger that causes aggressive actions. Where are you on your anger ladder? The higher on your ladder, the more unstable you are. Your goal is to keep your feet on solid ground. The best time to get control is on the bottom rung.

Watch for physical signs of anger. If you have trouble identifying anger until you are way up on your anger ladder, watch for physical changes in your body that may indicate you are angry, such as a rapid heartbeat, faster breathing, tension in your body (i.e., clenched hands or jaw), restlessness, pacing, shaking your leg, tapping of feet or hands, sweating, or trembling.

> ### Questions to Ponder
> Keep track of your anger this week. Answer the questions about your anger experiences:
>
> 28.1) What physical symptoms accompany your anger? Where are you on your anger ladder when you notice these symptoms?
>
> 28.2) What experiences or circumstances triggered your anger?
>
> 28.3) Use the following calming strategies this week. Which works best for you?

Keep Calm: Fast-acting strategies to use in the heat of the moment

Respond, don't react

Take a timeout. This strategy involves stepping away until you can handle the situation well. Leave, if possible, or stop the discussion until a later time. Stop, relax, and think so you can respond well instead of reacting in anger.

Preempt your anger. Prepare ahead of time if there is a likelihood that addressing a conflict may end with one or both people involved losing control of their anger. Agree, before emotions get out of control, that either person may call a time-out to pause the conversation and finish the discussion later. This gives both people time to deal with anger, preventing escalation.

Relax and breathe

The fastest way to calm down is to **focus on your breathing**. Deep breathing from your diaphragm causes a physical change, which calms your body and mind. Be aware that chest breathing does not work. You need to inhale from the deepest part of your gut and visualize all the stress leaving your body as you exhale. Exhale slowly, for longer than the inhale. If it helps, imagine a peaceful place while breathing.

Exercise — Push a wall

Physical exertion relieves tension in your body. Clean your house, go for a walk, or lift weights at the gym. Anger causes energy, and getting that energy out of your body clears your mind to deal with the anger. **Do not hit** a pillow or punching bag, as this may have the opposite effect. A fight response is created in your mind when you hit objects, feeding your body with even more energy.

One effective method for releasing the energy from anger is to push a wall. Walk up to a **sturdy** wall or doorframe. Do not run, as you may push right through it! Place your hands on the wall and your feet away from it, as if you are trying to push the wall down. Push as hard as you can; yell at the wall if you want. The goal is to push on the wall until your arms and legs grow weak and you physically cannot push any more. Release all the angry energy from your body onto the wall. Then you will have the ability to process what angered you and how to handle the situation.

Healthy Processing of Anger

Anger makes it difficult to keep from saying or doing the wrong thing, so in a moment of anger, stop and be **SILENT**. Once you have calmed down, you can process what you are feeling.

Use the S.I.L.E.N.T strategy that follows to help process anger and avoid aggressive behaviors

> ## Questions to Ponder
> Read the following S.I.L.E.N.T. strategy and put it into practice.
>
> **28.4) Write about using the strategy.**
>
> **28.5) How did the strategy help you?**
>
> **28.6) Where did you find the strategy difficult to implement?**

Strategy: S.I.L.E.N.T.

Stop

Catching anger right away is the key to managing it. Identify it, then take steps to clear your mind. Look for the physical signs of anger. When you first notice anger, take a time-out to walk, exercise, practice breathing or relaxation techniques, or talk with your coach or accountability partner.

Identify

Identify the cues or events that cause your hostility. Is the neighbor leaving trash in your yard or playing music too loud? Were you on hold too long, or did another's incompetence cause you to fail? Is someone stealing from you, or degrading you and spreading lies? What is the triggering event? What warning signs alert you to anger?

Look for the **physical cues** (i.e., bodily responses such as tight jaw or muscles, fast heart rate, surge of adrenalin, etc.), **behavioral cues** (glaring, raising your voice, etc.), **emotional cues** (other feelings like fear, hurt, jealousy, etc. that accompany or precede your anger), and **thought cues** (any thoughts that are increasing your hostility. Ask: Do I see images of aggression or have ideas of revenge?).

Ladder

Remember the anger ladder. Monitor your anger. If you struggle with severe anger issues, check your place on the anger ladder each morning and throughout the day. Write about it in your journal. Manage your anger on a moment-by-moment basis. Examine your cues and the related event and note the highest rung you climbed on the anger ladder. How are you bringing your feet back to ground level?

Explore

Explore the feelings and situations behind the anger. After you have identified the specific conflict, try to go further. What information can you learn from your anger? What about this situation caused you anger? Is a relationship unhealthy? Are you being mistreated, manipulated, or abused? Are you feeling inadequate or afraid of something? Do you want what you cannot have? How does this situation impact your life?

Negotiate

Negotiate the solution. Are you offended because of past experiences or assumptions? Is the perceived wrong legitimate? Are you being reasonable or taking something personally? What was your intent? Is it possible the other person did not intend harm or had a good motive? Should you resolve the conflict or deal with it in your heart? Discuss the issue with the person involved in love.

Take

Take back your rights. You can resolve a conflict without allowing people to walk all over you. You have a legitimate right to be treated with respect and dignity. Conflict resolution always involves forgiving, but that does not mean you must put yourself in a position to continue suffering harm from another. Be assertive but not aggressive when standing up for yourself.

Chapter Ten

Anxiety & Fear Management

Lesson 29 — Anxiety

Everyone experiences fear—it is a normal emotion. Fear comes in many forms, including anxiety, jealousy, nervousness, insecurity, pride, or a strong, terrified response of panic. Like every other emotion, **fear gives you information**, alerting you to emotional or physical danger. If you listen to the information your fear provides, you will learn to navigate tough situations and avoid harmful situations.

Anxiety usually results from stress or worry—fear about what is happening or going to happen. Stress is normal and can occur in pleasant or unpleasant situations. It is normal to have some anxiety when preparing to give a speech, perform, or confront a difficult situation. Anxiety alerts you to the possibility of failure and urges caution. It tells you a situation is important and requires extra attention, or to prepare for a potentially negative response. Normal anxiety occurs in a known situation, circumstance, or environment, and it leaves when the stressor is no longer present.

Anxiety manifests in physical symptoms such as a clenched jaw, tight muscles in the neck and back, headaches, chest pain, rapid heartbeat, or shortness of breath. It can cause a physical sense of dread, often described as a knot in the pit of the stomach. Anxiety makes it difficult to concentrate; it causes you to spin up, becoming restless and "on edge."

> Because anxiety includes such an intense physical component, managing your physical symptoms first can help your mind process the thoughts causing your anxiety.

Problematic Anxiety

Anxiety that exists when there is no threat or danger and interferes with daily life may be the sign of an anxiety disorder. This form of anxiety is a response to a stressor that exists only in our thoughts. Sometimes we are not even aware of the thoughts or beliefs that trigger the anxiety.

Problematic anxiety is unsubstantiated, constant worry. It may cause you to avoid situations, fearing failure or the reactions of others. It may cause panic attacks seemingly without reason. Or it can manifest as an irrational fear or avoidance of a person, object, place, or situation that carries little or no threat of danger. Anxiety creates a need for control. One way an anxious mind tries to grasp control is with obsessive behaviors, such as Obsessive-Compulsive Disorder (OCD). Obsessive behaviors may include constant checking of things or excessive touching, arranging, or cleaning.

Anxiety creates anxiety. For someone with an anxiety disorder, just the prospect of having stress or experiencing a panic attack can cause or increase anxiety. People often cause themselves anxiety by inventing self-defeating beliefs to escape their sense of dread.

Questions to Ponder

29.1) How do fear and anxiety affect your life?

29.2) Do you experience fear of social situations or other situations in which most people do not experience fear?

Anxiety without a Cause

Does it seem your anxiety has no origin or cause? This can happen with a **substance-induced anxiety disorder**, which occurs when anxiety symptoms develop from taking or stopping a drug. Alcohol, stimulants, caffeine, and some medications can cause an imbalance in the brain, which results in anxiety. Symptoms often cease within several weeks after the person stops using the substance.

Anxiety that originates from substance abuse affects a person's normal ability to cope with stressors, both new and old. Connecting substance-induced anxiety to past trauma can cause the symptoms to persist, even after the person ceases using the substance. If, however, anxiety was present before the use of a substance, it is not "substance-induced."

Suppressed emotions are another possible, hidden cause of anxiety. Many people cut off from their feelings because experiences have taught them that expressing emotion is wrong or even dangerous. People raised in an environment that did not allow them to understand or express their emotion often struggle with suppressed emotions.

Like anger, **anxiety is a common secondary emotion**; it is the emotion experienced instead of the suppressed emotion. If you cannot identify the situation that is making you anxious, it is possible there is an underlying emotion behind your anxiety. Many people who were raised without understanding emotions consider emotions weakness and reject them. People who do not express emotions well may experience anxiety in place of difficult emotions. The solution is learning to acknowledge and express your feelings and discover why you do not feel safe expressing the emotion.

Questions to Ponder

29.3) Do you experience anxiety resulting from taking, starting, or stopping an illegal drug, medication, or alcohol?

29.4) Are you able to express emotions such as grief, anger, pain, or sadness?

29.5) When do you consider it inappropriate to show emotions? When do you hide them?

29.6) If you struggle to express emotion, do you know why?

Fear leads us to want control, to protect ourselves. With anxiety, we try to control circumstances and situations around us, but in fact, **we can only control our own actions**.

The antidote to fear is trust in God, knowing yourself and God, and receiving His perfect love.

> *There is no fear in love, but perfect love casts out fear. For fear has to do with punishment, and whoever fears has not been perfected in love. (1 John 4:18)*
>
> *When I am afraid, I put my trust in you. (Psalm 56:3)*

Questions to Ponder

29.7) What situations are you still trying to control?

29.8) What is the fear behind your desire to control those situations?

29.9) Does your attempt at control alleviate the fear?

29.10) What different response to fear could you try that may lead to a better outcome?

Lesson 30 – Combat Anxiety & Panic Attacks

Anxiety disorders are a never-ending circle. Anxious thoughts lead to physical symptoms, which lead to behaviors that maintain and increase the anxiety.

Physical Anxiety Sensations

Anxious Thoughts

Anxiety-maintaining Behaviors

It starts with a thought or belief. Sometimes we experience the symptoms of anxiety first and are unaware of the thought or belief causing it. As a result, we assume our thoughts come from experiencing the emotion, but the truth is that the physical sensations we feel come from our thoughts.

We choose behaviors we expect will improve our anxiety, such as isolating from social scenes, attempting to take control, or avoiding challenging situations. These behaviors **lead to new beliefs**: We assume we are incapable or out of control. The new beliefs maintain or even increase the anxiety, and then this cycle repeats.

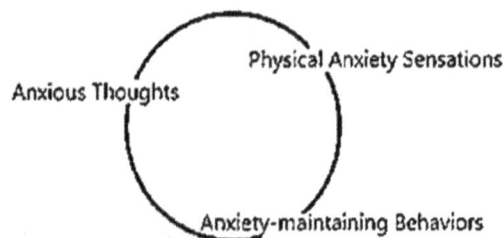

To break the cycle, you must break the chains of the circle using these three steps:

1. **Calm** the physical symptoms of anxiety. Live in the moment and use relaxation techniques.
2. **Challenge** your anxious thoughts and look for problematic thinking patterns.
3. **Discover and stop** the behaviors that maintain and worsen your anxiety, such as avoiding situations or criticizing yourself.

Truth You Can Trust In

God's perfect love casts out fear (see 1 John 4:18); His Word shows us truth that we can cling to when we experience anxiety and fear. Keep your mind focused on the truth in His Word.

- God gives us a spirit of power and self-control. Anxiety and fear are liars, tools of the enemy.
  FEAR: F – False **E** – Evidence **A** – Appearing **R** – Real

    For God gave us a spirit not of fear but of power and love and self-control. (2 Timothy 1:7)

- He will strengthen you to handle life's stressors.

    *Fear not, for I am with you; be not dismayed, for I am your God; I will strengthen you,
    I will help you, I will uphold you with my righteous right hand. (Isaiah 41:10)*

- He will supply your every need.

    *And my God will supply every need of yours according to his riches in glory in Christ Jesus.
    (Philippians 4:19)*

- He gives us a purpose and a future. We do not need to worry about the future.

    *For I know the plans I have for you, declares the LORD, plans for welfare and not for
    evil, to give you a future and a hope. (Jeremiah 29:11)*

    *Even to your old age I am he, and to gray hairs I will carry you.
    I have made, and I will bear; I will carry and will save. (Isaiah 46:4)*

- You can move on!

    *I press on toward the goal for the prize of the upward call of God in Christ Jesus.
    (Philippians 3:14)*

Strategy: R.E.A.S.O.N.

Trade in the chaos of anxiety for reason! We will have stressors in life. James 1:2 says to "Count it all joy, my brothers, when you meet trials of various kinds," but the one suffering with anxiety feels a need to control the trials instead of rejoicing in them. Learning to deal with anxiety in a healthy, biblical way **allows anxiety to work for you instead of controlling you.** *Remember the acrostic R.E.A.S.O.N. for dealing with anxiety:*

Relax

Relax your body and slow your breathing. Anxiety clouds your mind, preparing your body to fight or flee. This causes an adrenalin rush, rapid heartbeat, muscle tension, etc. Your body is not preparing your mind to think, but to take emergency action. By calming your physical response, you can clear your mind. (See the end of this chapter for relaxation tools.)

Examine

Examine your surroundings to help ground you in the moment. Stay in the here and now. Focus on an object in your hand, or do a task like washing dishes, and focus only on that task.

> *Therefore do not be anxious about tomorrow, for tomorrow will be anxious for itself.*
> *Sufficient for the day is its own trouble. (Matthew 6:34)*

Actual

Is there an actual threat or a real reason for your anxiety? Search your surroundings. Is there an external threat? What are the triggers?

Shift

Shift your mindset. Peace comes when your mind is stayed on the Lord. Meditate on the Word of the Lord and His truths; do not allow what you feel or see to deceive you.

> *You keep him in perfect peace whose mind is stayed on you, because he trusts in you. (Isaiah 26:3)*

> *Finally, brothers, whatever is true, whatever is honorable, whatever is just, whatever is pure, whatever is lovely, whatever is commendable, if there is any excellence, if there is anything worthy of praise, think about these things. (Philippians 4:8)*

Offer

Offer your burden to the Lord. Pray with gratitude in your heart for all God has done. It is difficult to worry about the future when you reflect on how the Lord has helped and blessed you in the past. Humble yourself and do not look to your own wisdom or try to take control. Give your anxieties to God and give Him the responsibility for the outcome.

> *Do not be anxious about anything, but in everything by prayer and supplication with thanksgiving let your requests be made known to God. (Philippians 4:6)*

> *Humble yourselves, therefore, under the mighty hand of God so that at the proper time he may exalt you, casting all your anxieties on him, because he cares for you. (1 Peter 5:6 – 7)*

New Thinking

Renew your mind and think differently. Changing how you process information involves seeking truth and rejecting messages that reinforce insecurity, pain, shame, and fear from past situations. Seek wisdom to discern truth from the problematic thinking prompting your anxiety.

> *If any of you lacks wisdom, let him ask God, who gives generously to all without reproach, and it will be given him. (James 1:5)*

Calming and Relaxation

With anxiety, your clouded mind makes relaxation difficult. Employing simple techniques to help clear your mind and calm physical sensations will give you the ability to handle anxiety and panic. For people who experience anxiety daily, the body adapts to the nervous, jittery feelings, and this becomes the new normal for them. Over time, intentional relaxation can reduce the amount of tension the body considers "normal."

Be careful not to use relaxation techniques as an excuse not to deal with the underlying issues causing your anxiety. This is a danger of this technique. When you feel and function better, it is easier to fall into avoidance rather than to deal with what is making you uncomfortable.

You may be tempted to skip relaxation exercises unless you are experiencing extreme anxiety or panic, but this is also a mistake. **Using relaxation only to stop panic, rather than using it to prevent panic, sends a message to your brain that anxiety is bad.** Anxiety is a normal emotion that everyone experiences in response to a perceived threat. When your brain treats anxiety as the threat, any moment that would trigger normal anxiety creates a strong anxious response. Your mind is responding to dual threats: the trigger and the anxiety. **It is as if you become afraid to fear.**

Relax Safely

Use the following guidelines for relaxation as a **preemptive**, routine practice. Treat relaxation as exercise. The more you do it, the stronger you get at it. Make relaxation part of your daily routine. Be intentional. Set time aside to relax in the morning, and before and after stressful situations. This will help you cope with life instead of avoiding it. These transformational techniques are so simple that you can do them anywhere, and they only take a few minutes.

Questions to Ponder

Read the REASON strategy and put it into practice.

30.1) Write about using the strategy.

30.2) How did the strategy help you?

30.3) Where did you find the strategy difficult to implement?

30.4) How do you relax? Write the ways you currently relax.

30.5) How often do you spend time relaxing?

30.6) What activities do you enjoy that your anxiety prevents you from doing?

30.7) Try the relaxation techniques that follow. How do you feel about using these techniques?

Slow your body down to help your mind get through difficult episodes of anxiety.

For God alone, O my soul, wait in silence, for my hope is from him. (Psalm 62:5)

Relaxation Techniques

Just Breathe — Rectangle

1. Breathe in from your diaphragm, not your chest. Fold your hands on your belly and notice your belly fill with air.

2. Do not take extra deep breaths. The point is to slow your breathing, not take in more air.

3. Picture a rectangle in your mind. Breathe in slowly to the count of five as you follow an imaginary rectangle in your mind.

4. Hold your breath to the count of three. Exhale slowly to the count of five and then hold to the count of three. Continue to follow the rectangle in your mind.

5. Repeat for about 10 minutes. Do this exercise each morning, evening, and when a situation overwhelms you, before the anxiety becomes severe.

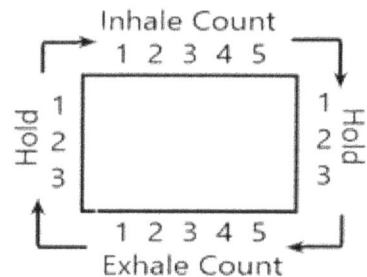

Inhale Count
1 2 3 4 5
Hold 1 2 3
Hold 1 2 3
1 2 3 4 5
Exhale Count

Slow Your Mind

Racing thoughts accompany anxiety. When your mind spins up, guided by unclear thoughts, it creates pressure to act. When your efforts to regain control of your mind fail, anxiety increases. Realize it is not possible to stop a thought from entering your mind. The problem is not your thought, but what you do with it. **A thought is just a thought.** It can be truth or a lie, but it cannot hurt you. **You need not act on the thought or control it.** When anxiety comes, observe your thoughts and let the anxiety pass through you and out of you like a wave; ride the wave to dry ground.

Ride the wave:

1. **Relax.** Tense and relax each muscle in your body one at a time until your entire body relaxes, notice the thoughts and sensations of anxiety flowing through and out of you like a wave.

2. **Do you feel safe?** God is your safe place. Secure yourself in the Lord. When you know you are in a safe place, you can observe your thoughts without interacting with them.

3. **Self-talk.** Remind yourself that nothing is going to hurt you and that this wave will end. If you can identify a specific thought, take it captive and focus on how the Lord's truth applies to it.

4. **Redirect your thoughts.** Do an activity or focus on something tangible. For example, hold a cold glass in your hand, focusing on the temperature of the glass, the texture, the size. Concentrate on the solid ground underneath each step you take. Do a chore like dishes, focusing on the water texture, the cloth, the motion of the towel, and so on.

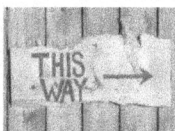

Self-care is vital to recovery from anxiety. This includes good sleep, good diet, exercise, setting goals, relating well with others, and doing activities you enjoy. If anxiety interferes with your ability to live a productive life, **ask your coach for additional resources**.

115

Lesson 31 — A Completed Inventory

A New "Heart Check Plan"

Progress Check and New Goals

You have completed the inventory of your past and examined patterns in your thoughts and actions. You may see how one event from your life set the stage for other events. Most likely, this information has changed how you think about your life, yourself, and God, and influenced a different way of dealing with situations.

Look at the "Heart Check Plan" that you created before starting your inventory. What progress have you made towards achieving your goals? Have your goals changed?

_____

_____

_____

_____

_____

_____

Make New Goals or Write the Goals You Are Still Working Toward

List the areas you wish to correct

For each item you wish to correct, write the result you want to see.

Introduction to Book Three

Relationship with God

Having a relationship with God is vital to our faith. It is through relationship that we learn to understand the God we follow and know ourselves as individuals created in His image. It is only through our relationship with God that we can grasp who we are, identify lies about ourselves, and understand our purpose. Having a right relationship with God allows us to have healthy relationships with people and brings us to a place of biblical love for self. Confidence in God can give us confidence in ourselves—something we often lack.

To have confidence in yourself, you need to know the true source of your worth and value. In the last book, you took a step toward knowing yourself by examining what is in your heart. But to truly grasp your identity, you must know God. That will be the focus of this book.

In This Book

Blessings & Gratitude

In this chapter, you will learn how to change your focus from negative things in your life and discover how the Lord uses them for good, and you will learn to recognize hidden blessings.

Restoration

This chapter will focus on making amends and forgiving others. This helps put us in a right relationship with the Lord, releasing us from the burden of guilt and need for retribution, and relieving the pain in our heart for good.

Purpose

Your appreciation for life changes as you discover purpose and value through our God. This allows your confidence for your future to grow. You should not ask whether you are able. The real question is, do you believe God can make you able?

Loving Who You Are in Christ

You are worth everything God has for you because He has made you worthy. In this chapter, you will learn how you cannot love God or others without loving yourself. You will learn the difference between humility and living in humiliation. You will love the person God created you to be!

Identifying & Removing Lies

Who does God say you are? What is the truth you should hold, in contrast to the lies and labels you have been carrying through life? You are not what you do. You are not your past, your failures, or your mistakes. You are not the labels others have placed on you or the labels you place on yourself. So who are you? Do you trust the report of the Lord, which is truth and leads to life, or are you deceived by the report of the enemy, a lie that leads to death? Whose report will you believe?

Chapter Eleven

Blessings & Gratitude

Lesson 32 — Blessings

Serve the L<small>ORD</small> with gladness! Come into his presence with singing! Know that the L<small>ORD</small>, he is God! It is he who made us, and we are his; we are his people, and the sheep of his pasture. Enter his gates with thanksgiving, and his courts with praise! Give thanks to him; bless his name! For the L<small>ORD</small> is good; his steadfast love endures forever, and his faithfulness to all generations. (Psalm 100: 2 – 5)

The Lord Makes Your Life a Blessing!

For I consider that the sufferings of this present time are not worth comparing with the glory that is to be revealed to us. (Romans 8:18)

In our inventory, we give a lot of attention to the negative things that happened in our lives. Here we look at how the Lord has used these situations to our good, and we recognize hidden blessings.

Rejoice always, pray without ceasing, give thanks in <u>all circumstances</u>; for this is the will of God in Christ Jesus for you. (1 Thessalonians 5:16 – 18)

It is easy to praise God when things are going well, but it is more difficult to praise Him in trials, pain, loss, and suffering. How do you react to life's difficulties? How do you respond to people failing you? Are you grateful through painful circumstances or when suffering loss?

Through him then let us continually offer up a <u>sacrifice of praise</u> to God, that is, the fruit of lips that acknowledge his name. (Hebrews 13:15)

I will offer to you the <u>sacrifice of thanksgiving </u>and call on the name of the L<small>ORD</small>. (Psalm 116:17)

Scripture calls our praise a sacrifice. What makes gratitude and thanksgiving a sacrifice? The Hebrew word used for sacrifice is *zabach*, which means to slaughter. This raises the question: What does gratitude slaughter?

Praising the Lord slaughters self and destroys pride. When you give our gratitude to the Lord, you are sacrificing boasting in yourself to boast in Him. Gratitude sacrifices your right to self-pity. You must give up your attitude of grumbling and complaining, taking your attention off self, circumstance, and your right to "vent." Giving thanks slaughters our flesh to set our hearts on the goodness of the Lord. It is not possible to wallow in misery when you are praising the Lord.

Enter his gates with thanksgiving, and his courts with praise! Give thanks to him; bless his name! (Psalm 100:4)

Do not be anxious about anything, but in everything by prayer and supplication <u>with thanksgiving </u>let your requests be made known to God. (Philippians 4:6 – 7)

Do all things without grumbling or disputing. (Philippians 2:14)

Try this brief experiment

In your mind, say the alphabet and count to twenty simultaneously. It cannot be done. You may go back and forth between numbers and letters with super speed, but your **conscious mind** cannot think of both at the exact same moment. It is not possible to consider two thoughts at once, proving that while you are reflecting on praiseworthy things, negativity cannot inhabit your conscious thoughts.

The Mind of Christ

> *For who has understood the mind of the Lord so as to instruct him?*
> *But we have the mind of Christ. (1 Corinthians 2:16)*

Fill your mind with God's word. Fix your eyes on Him, and even in the most trying situations, you will see hope, truth, and a future of promise. **Negativity, fear, and worry are the fruit of a world deprived of God.**

God is good; He wills only good, and He works all things together for the good of those who love Him. He never has a gloomy outlook. **Therefore, a gloomy outlook does not unify us with God's mind and will.** God working all things for good means everything, even bad things, are beneficial for the believer. If you receive a situation as negative, you are not seeing it the way the Lord does. You have a corrupted perspective.

Negative thoughts are void of God's Word. The solution is more than attempting to speak God's Word into a circumstance to alter its outcome. It is knowing **God's mind** regarding your situations. It is **believing that truth and His purposes prevail** through every inconvenience and trial and in our lives. This is what it means to "fight the good fight of faith."

> A Christian's confidence is knowing that God moves in everything.
> A life surrendered, walking with God, cannot fail.

Identify Negativity

When you react to situations with worry, or have concern about the opinions or responses of others, are you trusting the Lord? Reactions that are fearful or riddled with anger and negativity show a place in your life where the truth of God's Word has not yet penetrated. **Use your negative thoughts and doubt** to discover areas devoid of His Word, to motivate your prayers, and to guide you into a deeper relationship with and greater trust of Him.

Questions to Ponder

32.1) In what situations or areas of your life do you have a poor response? Where is there negativity in your thoughts?

32.2) How can you apply God's Word to the situations you identified?

32.3) Consider your negative situations, outlooks, and thoughts. In which areas do you recognize a need to grow in trust of the Lord?

32.4) How can you give praise to God in these situations?

32.5) In what areas are you still resentful of God? Where do you find it impossible to recognize anything good?

Lesson 33 — Seeing Life through New Eyes

At times, it is difficult to find God in life's trials. Have you ever wondered, "Where was God when I needed Him?" Scripture claims He **is** there, helping us overcome. The Lord does not hurt us, but sometimes His healing feels painful. Think of it as if you were going to the doctor with a broken bone. The doctor did not cause the injury, but for proper healing, he must rebreak and reset the bone. Likewise, the Lord does not cause our suffering, but the rebreaking required for healing can be painful.

He heals the brokenhearted and binds up their wounds. (Psalm 147:3)

For he wounds, but he binds up; he shatters, but his hands heal. (Job 5:18)

Why Do We Have Troubles?

Do you sometimes find it hard to understand why there is so much suffering in the world? Nowhere does Scripture say we will have an easy life. In fact, the Word tells us we enter God's Kingdom through trial and tribulation; but it also says the Lord will be with us in it.

Strengthening the souls of the disciples, encouraging them to continue in the faith, and saying that through many tribulations we must enter the kingdom of God.
(Acts 14:22)

Tests of faith strengthen us and increase our ability to persevere. Our weakness is the best display of God's power. Seeing the Lord work through difficulty teaches us to trust Him more.

Beloved, do not be surprised at the fiery trial when it comes upon you to test you, as though something strange were happening to you. (1 Peter 4:12)

So that the tested genuineness of your faith—more precious than gold that perishes though it is tested by fire—may be found to result in praise and glory and honor at the revelation of Jesus Christ. (1 Peter 1:7)

The enemy is not the only cause of our trials. Sometimes our flesh or other people's bad choices are the cause, and sometimes the Lord tests us. Whatever the cause, **God never wastes a situation or trial.** He uses it all to **keep us humble and transform our character.** The difficult things in life help us to grow. A test may come a short time after a victory, to strengthen an area we have overcome. The purpose is to go deeper into victory until we receive wholeness and perfection, standing firm in the Lord.

So to keep me from becoming conceited because of the surpassing greatness of the revelations, a thorn was given me in the flesh, a messenger of Satan to harass me, to keep me from becoming conceited. (2 Corinthians 12:7)

Count it all joy, my brothers, when you meet trials of various kinds, for you know that the testing of your faith produces steadfastness. And let steadfastness have its full effect, that you may be perfect and complete, lacking in nothing. (James 1:2 – 4)

125

The Lord uses hard situations to teach us about Him and His ways. He uses trials to show us truth, teach, and guide us, but He is gentle and disciplines us in love.

It is good for me that I was afflicted, that I might learn your statutes. (Psalm 119:71)

For the Lord disciplines the one he loves and chastises every son whom he receives.
(Hebrews 12:6)

How we handle trials may be an opportunity to make God known to the lost. When hardship weakens us, God's power is demonstrated in our lives.

I want you to know, brothers, that what has happened to me has really served
to advance the gospel, so that it has become known throughout the whole
imperial guard and to all the rest that my imprisonment is for Christ. And most
of the brothers, having become confident in the Lord by my imprisonment, are
much more bold to speak the word without fear.
(Philippians 1:12 – 14)

For the sake of Christ, then, I am content with weaknesses, insults, hardships,
persecutions, and calamities. For when I am weak, then I am strong.
(2 Corinthians 12:9 – 10)

Trials may come simply because we follow Christ. Scripture says that a believer will share in the sufferings of Christ. The world will hate us for His name's sake, and we will suffer persecution, revilement, and false accusations. But Scripture also says that we have a glorious reward for our suffering.

Blessed are those who are persecuted for righteousness' sake, for theirs is the kingdom
of heaven. Blessed are you when others revile you and persecute you and utter all kinds
of evil against you falsely on my account. Rejoice and be glad, for your reward is great in
heaven, for so they persecuted the prophets who were before you.
(Matthew 5:10 – 12)

God rewards us as we persevere and helps us overcome our suffering. **When God enters our mess**, He brings us through, and healing happens!

Many are the afflictions of the righteous, but the Lord underlined delivers him out of them all.
(Psalm 34:19)

And after you have suffered a little while, the God of all grace, who has called you to his
eternal glory in Christ, will himself restore, confirm, strengthen, and establish you.
(1 Peter 5:10)

The one who conquers and who keeps my works until the end, to him I
will give authority over the nations.
(Revelation 2:26)

A God's Eye View of Your Life

When you look past your pain and discover the truth of Scripture in your trials, you will recognize the magnificence of the Lord. Only the Lord can show you His perspective on the events in your life. **The following tips and questions may aid your search for God's truth.**

- First, always test your beliefs against Scripture. If your thoughts do not line up with the **whole of Scripture**, they are not correct.

- Seek the Lord for His wisdom. Be open to hearing truth; the Lord will give understanding.

- Find the benefit resulting from the circumstance. What is the report of the Lord?

Questions to Ponder

33.1) Reexamine your heart check and inventory lists from God's perspective. Answer all six questions for each item mentioned in your inventory lists.

1. What did you learn? What did the trial expose about your character?
2. How was your faith tested?
3. How did your character grow from the experience, or how could it have grown?
4. How has the situation brought you to rely on God or increase your faith?
5. How has God kept you from a greater harm in the situation?
6. How has God improved your life or character (or the life or character of another) by allowing this to happen?

33.2) What good do you see from your trials? How can you give praise to God for the trials you have experienced in your life?

33.3) Write all the good and praises from the above answers in your Blessings Journal. *(Reference the homework below.)*

> ➢ **Begin a new "Blessings Journal"** to keep a record of what the Lord has done in your journey and for your life.
> ➢ **When you feel negative and discouraged, this journal will remind you of God's truth and provision.**
> ➢ **Pray your praises to the Lord!**

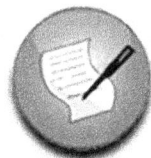

Chapter Twelve

Restoration

Lesson 34 — Forgiveness

During your inventory in Book Two, you found times that you hurt people, and times people hurt you. Although you gave your past pain to the Lord, **complete freedom** from anger, guilt, and fear requires that you release unforgiveness in your heart and make amends for your wrongs.

We will begin with forgiveness. Why start there? Sometimes, looking at your resentments toward others allows you to recognize your own wrongs. These situations may help you discover amends you need to make (though this is not always the case).

> ## Questions to Ponder
> **34.1) Define forgiveness. In your understanding, what does it mean to forgive someone?**

Forgiveness Is Not …

Do you struggle to understand forgiveness? Society distorts the meaning, making true, biblical forgiveness a hard concept to grasp.

Do you find yourself replaying certain situations over and over in your mind, or do you feel like you must forgive someone repeatedly **for the same transgression**? If so, you may misunderstand forgiveness. Scripture commands believers to forgive, but many have no clue what that means. People often believe forgiveness means accepting someone's apology and not bringing the matter back up. This is not the definition of forgiveness. This cannot eliminate your pain; instead, it masks it. You need not forgive the **same event** multiple times. True forgiveness happens once per offense.

One common definition of forgiveness is a **decision to release resentful feelings** toward another who has harmed you, without condoning, excusing, or forgetting their wrong. Yet this definition is lacking. **How do you release resentful feelings without getting justice?** This definition bases forgiveness on **feelings**. With this notion of forgiveness, you create an **obligation** in your mind to no longer experience anger, even if it is entirely reasonable to have anger about a situation. **In reality, you are not forgetting the offense; you are attempting to forget what you** *feel* **about the offense.**

If your attempts at forgiving are ending resentment, you are probably understanding forgiveness in this way. Any trigger that reminds you of the wrong done to you brings back pain, and then you need to forgive again. It may take years for the resentment in your heart to dissipate, and this can cause a deeper, **repressed** resentment because you are pushing pain aside instead of addressing it.

Forgiveness Is …

Let us look at what is true in the false ideas of forgiveness discussed above. **Forgiveness is a choice** you make, but true forgiveness releases pain and resentment. You do not forget the offense, nor condone the wrong behavior. **Real forgiveness is a decision, not to release resentment, but to offer forgiveness**. People misunderstand forgiveness **because they do not understand the choice** they are making.

Releasing resentment is not forgiveness, rather is the result of forgiving.

The Greek biblical word for forgiveness is ***aphesis,*** which means dismissal, release, or pardon. We know a person should "pay" for harm they cause, and we have a right to justice. The demand in our heart for justice creates a burden of resentment and anger until restitution is made. **But it is also our God-given right to remedy the debt owed for harm another caused. Forgiveness is the remedy that cancels the debt.**

Consider a loan forgiveness program. The program "forgives" the owed debt and thereby cancels the debt. The lender can no longer ask you for the money because **the debt no longer exists**. It cleared as if paid in full, and the lender will never bring it back up again. The lender does not carry around a burden, waiting for the day you pay your debt.

In a similar way, actual forgiveness releases our right to retribution by giving the Lord our right to remedy the debt owed to us. This takes away our resentment as well. The Lord carries the burden of our retribution. **Collecting on the debt becomes His responsibility, and it is over for us.**

God wants this responsibility. Our sense of justice is corrupted by our emotions and sin nature. When we are harmed, we sometimes feel the consequence pales in comparison to the pain a person caused, wanting them to suffer more for their offense. When we are the offender, our efforts to resolve issues are sometimes lacking and disingenuous.

Because God is just, His forgiveness is based on the actions of the one needing forgiveness, but **our forgiveness cannot depend upon the actions of the one who hurt us**. Only God can remove a person's sin, and only His retribution is just. If the offender repents and comes to the Lord, He is right to forgive the offense. We can trust the Lord will work to bring the offender to repentance, and if they refuse, we can trust the Lord to handle it. **Either way**, **our forgiveness guarantees justice.**

> *The Rock, his work is perfect, for all his ways are justice. A God of faithfulness and without iniquity, just and upright is he. (Deuteronomy 32:4)*

Forgiveness

God Himself models forgiveness for us. When we repent or turn away from our sin, He is faithful to forgive. Sin requires a penalty, and Jesus paid that debt. The wage of sin is death. **Jesus is like the loan forgiveness program that cancels our sin debt.** Our lives are the price we owe for our sins. **We pay the debt, one way or another.** If we decide to continue in sin, we pay the debt eternally. If we give our lives to the Lord, Jesus pays the price for us.

> *For the wages of sin is death, but the free gift of God is eternal life in Christ Jesus our Lord.*
> *(Romans 6:23)*

> *The sting of death is sin, and the power of sin is the law.*
> *(1 Corinthians 15:56)*

When we repent, the Lord separates us from our sin as far as the east is from the west, and He remembers it no more. Our debt collector no longer has the right to harass us, and sin loses its condemning power. When God forgives, He does not "forget" our sin; **He no longer remembers it.** What is the difference? God knows we committed the sin, but when he forgives, He no longer brings it to His memory to rehash or act on it. **God does not dwell on our past mistakes, and neither should we.** He helps us correct our mistakes and move forward. A sin forgiven is over. We need not continue to ask God's forgiveness for past wrongs.

Likewise, when we forgive someone for their wrongs to us, we do not need to remember or dwell on their sin. Yes, we know what happened, but we trust the Lord to make it right, and it opens the door to **restoration** of the relationship, *if the person is repentant* for their wrongs.

> *For I will be merciful toward their iniquities, and I will remember their sins no more.*
> *(Hebrews 8:12)*

> *As far as the east is from the west, so far does he remove our transgressions from us.*
> *(Psalm 103:12)*

Why Forgive?

➤ We forgive because we are forgiven.

> *Put on then, as God's chosen ones, holy and beloved, compassionate hearts, kindness, humility, meekness, and patience, bearing with one another and, if one has a complaint against another, forgiving each other; <u>as the Lord has forgiven you, so you also must forgive.</u>*
> *(Colossians 3:12 – 13)*

➤ As we forgive others is how we are forgiven.

> *For if you forgive others their trespasses, your heavenly Father will also forgive you, but if you do not forgive others their trespasses, neither will your Father forgive your trespasses.*
> *(Matthew 6:14 – 15)*

> *And whenever you stand praying, forgive, if you have anything against anyone, so that your Father also who is in heaven may forgive you your trespasses. (Mark 11:25)*

> *Judge not, and you will not be judged; condemn not, and you will not be condemned; forgive, and you will be forgiven. (Luke 6:37)*

> *Then his master summoned him and said to him, "You wicked servant! I forgave you all that debt because you pleaded with me. And should not you have had mercy on your fellow servant, as I had mercy on you?" And in anger his master delivered him to the jailers, until he should pay all his debt. So also my heavenly Father will do to every one of you, if you do not forgive your brother from your heart. (Matthew 18:32 – 35)*

➤ We are all sinners needing forgiveness.

> *If we say we have no sin, we deceive ourselves, and the truth is not in us. (1 John 1:8)*

➤ We forgive repeat offenses.

> *Then Peter came up and said to him, "Lord, how often will my brother sin against me, and I forgive him? As many as seven times?" Jesus said to him, "I do not say to you seven times, but seventy times seven." (Matthew 18:21 – 22)*

The Heart of Forgiveness

Scripture tells us that forgiveness is a genuine act of love. We are to love our enemies. Forgiveness begins with **pity**. What is the other person's situation? Pity for another does not excuse their actions; it is empathy for the pain in their hearts, which led them to hurt us. If we can understand the pain another has gone through, it is a step toward forgiving them.

Having a heart of **gratitude** makes it possible to forgive even devastating harm. If you are grateful for good resulting from a situation, forgiveness comes more easily. If you are grateful for the forgiveness you have received, it is easier to forgive another.

How Do I Forgive?

First, look at the harm and understand the situation. This does not justify another's actions, but it removes some of the emotional sting, allowing you to consider the whole picture.

> Start by asking yourself these questions:
>> What was the actual harm done?
>> Was the wrong intentional? What happened to cause the person to act that way? Is there room for pity?
>> Were their hurtful words or actions a response to something I did or said?
>> Was I correct in my handling of the situation? Were there wrongs on both sides?

> Next, release the offender from their debt of retribution.
>> Give it to the Lord and ask Him to take your pain and resentment. Allow the burden of justice to fall on His shoulders and not yours.

> Finally, expect God to be faithful and just, knowing that justice happens in His timing and may not be instantaneous.

Remember, **God is as patient with others as He is with you**. Have confidence that justice will come. If the offender repents and changes his way, then justice has come. If he does not repent, the Lord administers His justice. Either way, your pain is vindicated.

When Do I Forgive?

You should forgive as soon as possible. Otherwise, hurt festers inside and builds resentment in your heart. Forgiveness is for your freedom as much as, or more, than it is for the person you forgive.

Restoration

Forgiveness is not restoration. These are two separate things. To restore a relationship with someone requires that both parties understand the problem and walk in agreement. This is especially true when the person **continues to cause you the same harm**.

Reconciliation comes after a person shows repentance. Remember, repentance means the person changes how they treat you. **You can** forgive someone who is **not** repentant. However, you should **not restore a damaging relationship** that continues to hurt you. Restoration should happen only after the person repents. Reconciliation often requires rebuilding a relationship from a healthy starting point, or else the same harmful situations could repeat.

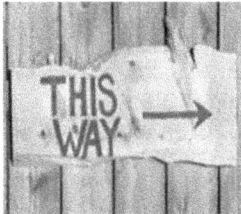

Make no effort at contact if harm could come to you or another person. It is not always necessary to tell someone you forgave them.

Ask your coach if you are unsure whether you should contact an offender or restore a relationship with someone.

Your coach is **not** permitted to tell you what to do in any given situation, but he or she may have additional insight that can help you make a wise decision.

Questions to Ponder

34.2) Do you understand forgiveness better since reading this lesson? Explain, in your own words, what forgiveness means, and how to forgive another.

34.3) Do you still hold resentment and unforgiveness toward anyone?

34.4) Write a letter to each person you need to forgive. Explain their actions and how you want to release them. *Do not give them the letters.* They are only meant to be a step to help you process your feelings.

34.5) Forgive any offenders and pray, giving the situation to the Lord. Give Him your burden, pain, and resentment. Relinquish your right to retribution to His perfect judgment and put your justice in His hands.

The next book goes into more detail about
restoring relationships and dealing with conflict.

Lesson 35 — Making Amends for Wrongs

In this lesson, you will examine and make amends for the wrongs you have done to others. Before you can confess your wrongs to another or to God, **you must admit them to yourself**.

> ### Questions to Ponder
> During your inventory, you made a list of people you have harmed by your words or actions. Has this list grown? Is there guilt in your heart not addressed in your list?
>
> **35.1) Add to your list any additional harms or recent harms you may have caused.**

Confess to Another and God

After identifying your wrongs, confess them. If you have not already done so, take the harms you caused others to your coach and pray for the Lord's forgiveness. Then your heart will be ready to make a genuine amends to the person whom you hurt if this is possible.

Why Should I Admit My Mistakes?

You may think because you did wrong years ago, there is no longer a reason to admit the mistake. Perhaps your actions cause you shame. No one wants to have to say, "I was wrong." For some people, admitting fault is terribly difficult. Yet making amends for your past wrongs is one of the most healing steps of your journey, not only for you, but also for the one to whom you apologize. We can never realize the full impact of our words and actions. Your apology may heal deep pain in a person's heart.

Admitting mistakes releases a burden from your shoulders that you may not even know you carry. It is a humbling experience, freeing you from the weight of guilt and regret. The heaviness of your secret sins lifts as you expose your wrongs to the light.

For when I kept silent, my bones wasted away through my groaning all day long. For day and night your hand was heavy upon me; my strength was dried up as by the heat of summer.
(Psalm 32:3 – 4)

Therefore, confess your sins to one another and pray for one another, that you may be healed. The prayer of a righteous person has great power as it is working.
(James 5:16)

What Does It Mean to Make Amends?

Making amends means taking responsibility for your wrong and attempting to make it right. Most often this is done with a letter or email containing a sincere, written apology and an admission of wrongs. In certain situations, this can also be a phone call or face-to-face visit.

Amends **may involve more than an apology**, such as restoring, repairing, or replacing an item you stole or damaged. Righting your wrongs is a biblical concept. The Lord can forgive you, but He still wants you to make it right and reconcile, with the one you harmed, if possible.

134

So if you are offering your gift at the altar and there remember that your brother has something against you, leave your gift there before the altar and go. First be reconciled to your brother, and then come and offer your gift.
(Matthew 5:23 – 24)

If a man steals an ox or a sheep, and kills it or sells it, he shall repay five oxen for an ox, and four sheep for a sheep. (Exodus 22:1)

Whoever conceals his transgressions will not prosper, but he who confesses and forsakes them will obtain mercy. (Proverbs 28:13)

What If I Am Uncertain about My Wrongs?

You may encounter times when people accuse you of wrongdoing, **but you were not in the wrong**. People sometimes make assumptions about your intentions from your past mistakes or their own past hurts. They may feel wronged if they dislike your actions or choices, or if your behavior calls out their own issues and wounds. **You cannot change how people feel about you or your actions.**

Examine a circumstance where you disagree with a person's determination of your guilt to confirm if there was an actual wrong, or if it was the other person's issue. Before making amends, ask yourself, "Was I wrong for this action? Could different actions or words have caused less harm?" **You should make amends if you caused genuine harm to another, but do not accept blame that does not belong to you.** If you are not wrong, maintain your innocence.

People may be oversensitive to what you say or do because of their own insecurity, fears, or hurts. You **can and should** consider their feelings. While it is not okay to accept blame for their misunderstandings, you may ease their concerns if you **clarify your intent or feelings**.

Sometimes we are oblivious to the fact that our words or actions harmed a person. You cannot change what you do not know. It is not beneficial to worry about wrongs you are not sure you committed. Scripture is clear: **We are to make amends when we become aware of the sin or harm we caused.** Ask the Lord to show you any wrongs you have done, then repent, forgive, and make amends.

If anyone sins, doing any of the things that by the Lord's commandments ought not to be done, though he did not know it, <u>then realizes his guilt</u>, he shall bear his iniquity. He shall bring to the priest a ram without blemish out of the flock, or its equivalent, for a guilt offering, and the priest shall make atonement for him for the mistake that he made unintentionally, and he shall be forgiven. It is a guilt offering; he has indeed incurred guilt before the Lord.
(Leviticus 5:17 – 19)

Risks and Responsibilities

A good amends speaks about growth, how you came to understand your wrong, the reason for your regret, and what you did or will do to correct it. **A genuine amends never includes a "but."** "I am sorry for this, but you made me so angry." Apologies that dig at the one to whom you are apologizing, or that attempt to shift the blame, are not genuine.

There is a risk when you admit your faults to someone you harmed. Not everyone will accept your apology or offer you forgiveness. This is okay. **You are correcting a wrong, not soliciting a response.** Your amends should be unconditional. Never base an apology on a person's acceptance of it. Clarify that your amends have **no expectations** attached.

People may have expectations after you make amends. They may wish to remain distant when you desire restoration, or they may want to restore the relationship when you believe it is unhealthy. Amends **may** open a door to reconciliation, yet sometimes it is not in your best interest, or theirs, to restore the relationship. **An apology does not obligate you to commit yourself to a toxic relationship.**

There is always the risk that a recipient of your amends may reject you and your apology. People sometimes cannot get past their own hurt. They may believe you are toxic to them and choose separation. There are many reasons a person is unable to hear your apology with the loving intent in which you wrote it. Do everything in your power to be at peace, but prepare for rejection.

If possible, so far as it depends on you, live peaceably with all. (Romans 12:18)

It is important to consider the possibility of harm from contacting a person. If it is possible that your amends will cause harm to you or others, **do not** approach the person. For example, a person may be unaware of the harm you caused, such as if you had judgmental or wrong thoughts about them. In this or any situation in which you cannot give an amends letter to the person you have wronged; you should still write the letter. Repent of your wrong thoughts or actions but share the amends letter only with God and your coach. Ask God's forgiveness and seek His wisdom about sharing the amends with the one harmed. Consult with your coach if you are unsure.

Questions to Ponder

35.2) Have you asked the Lord for forgiveness for all your wrongs? If not, do so now.

35.3) Are you prepared to express your regret for the harm you have caused?

35.4) Who may be harmed by your amends? Think about relationships that your letter might affect—*yourself, the one you harmed*, a *spouse, child, etc.*

35.5) Are there ways besides an apology to rectify some of your wrongs, such as restoring
or replacing something you took or damaged? If yes, list them.

35.6) Write a letter to each person to whom you need to make amends. Explain what you did to them, how you realized your wrong, and why you want to make it right.

   1. Explain that you have no expectation of a response to the letter. It is a no-strings-attached apology.

   2. Do not shift the blame. You are making an apology for your wrongs, not addressing their wrongs. Your apology should include no "but" statements.

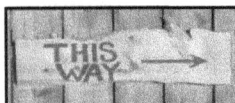

THIS WAY → Do not approach someone, even by letter, if giving them an amends could cause you or another harm or put you in danger.

Chapter Thirteen

Purpose

Lesson 36 — Identity & Purpose

Have you ever wondered about your identity or purpose? Reading the Bible and calling on the Holy Spirit can help you discover your unique identity, purpose, and worth in Christ. The scriptures are more than generic statements for all followers; **they are specific to you**!

We have a future. We have an eternal purpose. We have hope. We have value.

Questions to Ponder

36.1) Do you struggle with knowing your identity in Christ? If yes, how?

36.2) Do you struggle to identify what makes you unique or special? Explain.

36.3) Do you struggle to know where you belong or to find a place to feel you "fit"?

36.4) What gives you value? Do you struggle to find your worth?

36.5) What do you believe is your purpose in life?

What Your Purpose Is NOT

Your purpose is not the "pursuit of happiness." **Happiness should not be a measure of success or value.** When you pursue the Lord's purpose for your life, **the result** includes happiness, but when your pursuit in life is merely to live happy, safe, and worry-free, you will find it to be a miserable existence. It is the trials in life—the sad moments and grief—which teach compassion, love, and strength of character, and which give our lives depth and meaning. No one likes hard times, but those living life to avoid difficulties can be destroyed when a crisis or trial causes their safe, happy, secure life to fail them.

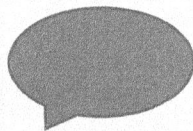

> "A life directed chiefly towards the fulfillment of personal desires will sooner or later always lead to bitter disappointment."
>
> Albert Einstein in a Letter to T. Lee, January 16, 1954

When what you are living for fails you, where is your hope? You may become anxious or depressed and need to redefine what it is that makes life worth living. You need hope based in the Lord for a successful future. Knowing your true purpose never leaves you disappointed. God has unique plans for you, and His promises to give you both hope and a future will never fail.

For I know the plans I have for you, declares the Lord, plans for welfare and not for evil, to give you a future and a hope. (Jeremiah 29:11)

Why Did God Create Us?

God was not lonely or vain when He created mankind, wanting someone to worship and adore Him. He did not desire servants or groundskeepers for the earth. God made the earth; He could care for it. God is not a control freak; He has every right to do as He wishes with His creation, **but He limited Himself** by giving us free will to make our own choices.

The God who made the world and everything in it, being Lord of heaven and earth, does not live in temples made by man, <u>nor is he served by human hands, as though he needed anything</u>, since he himself gives to all mankind life and breath and everything.
(Acts 17:24 – 25)

So, why *would* He need us? The answer speaks volumes.
God did *not* need us, He wanted us.

God created us to rule alongside Him. God's original intent for us is found in Genesis, when He created mankind **in His image and likeness** to fellowship and rule alongside Him.

Then God said, "Let us make man <u>in our image, after our likeness</u>. And let <u>them</u> <u>have dominion</u> over the fish … and over all the earth and over every creeping thing that creeps on the earth." (Genesis 1:26)

Do you not know that <u>we are to judge angels</u>? How much more, then, matters pertaining to this life! (1 Corinthians 6:3)

God created us to love us. "God is love" (1 John 4:8). Love, by definition, requires a recipient. God wants to overflow into us. God loved us even before we existed.

I have loved you with an everlasting love. (Jeremiah 31:3)

God created us for relationship with Him. The depth and intimacy of the relationship God desires is apparent all throughout Scripture in the relationship language he uses: "father," "children," "husband," "bride," etc. God wants to share life with us.

<u>For your Maker is your husband</u>, the Lord of hosts is his name; and the Holy One of Israel is your Redeemer, the God of the whole earth he is called.
(Isaiah 54:5)

Let us rejoice and exult and give him the glory, <u>for the marriage of the Lamb</u> has come, and his <u>Bride</u> has made herself ready.
(Revelation 19:7)

And because you are sons, God has sent the Spirit of his Son into our hearts, crying, "<u>Abba! Father!</u>"
(Galatians 4:6)

He created us to share a divine nature with Him. God offers us everything we need to restore the divine nature lost in the garden, preparing us for eternal life with Him. Saved, we are **becoming a new creation**, able **to partake in his divine nature** and escaping the world's corruption (our sin nature).

His divine power has granted to us all things that pertain to life and godliness, through the knowledge of him who called us to his own glory and excellence, by which he has granted to us his precious and very great promises, <u>so that through them you may</u> become <u>partakers of the divine nature</u>, having escaped from the corruption that is in the world because of sinful desire.
(2 Peter 1:3 – 4)

What does it mean to "share a divine nature" with God? The answer takes us back to Genesis. In the beginning God created man in His image and likeness. Adam and his wife shared God's image and were like Him, **but that does not mean they were gods.**

Adam and his wife walked in the garden with God, in His image, clothed in His Spirit, His glory resting on them. God gave them authority over all the earth, allowing them to rule next to Him as perfect creations with a free will. **They shared God's divine nature, the character and virtue that He possesses.** It is a nature **built on sacrificial love**, a nature **void of sin.**

Adam and his wife **traded in this divine nature for a sin nature** when they chose to disobey God. There were two trees prominently displayed in the center of the garden: the Tree of Life, and the Tree of the Knowledge of Good and Evil, which led to "death." From the beginning mankind was offered the same choice we are offered today. We can choose life and live in God's ways, or we can choose to operate in our own knowledge of good and evil, a path that leads to death. What died the day they ate? It wasn't their bodies. Rather, the nature of who they were created to be died that day. **They transformed into sinners.**

Christ's sacrifice gave mankind the ability to make the same choice. Choose life by choosing God and **be transformed back into Christ's likeness**, restoring the divine nature that was lost, or choose death, eternal separation from God, by rejecting God's wisdom for our flesh.

God is our source of life. All things are of Him and exist through Him. The first couple's disobedience separated all people from the Lord. Like a plant cut away from its root that decays and dies, humans were separated from God, their source, by the power of sin. Sin corrupted the entire earth: people, plants, and animals. Because of sin we get sick, our bodies break down, and we die.

Adam and Eve lost the likeness of God when they sinned, trading in their divine nature for a sin nature. Every person's DNA was in the first couple. When they fell, all of humanity fell with them, the seed corrupted. Therefore, the power of sin is at work in each of us from conception.

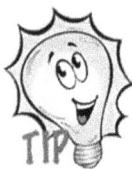

When we understand that we were created to be loved by God Himself, we can see that our **first purpose** is to have relationship with Christ. As that relationship grows, the Lord transforms our heart into His own likeness, restoring the likeness to the divine nature that was lost through sin. **This life is like boot camp training for our eternal purpose**, to rule and reign with Christ!

Questions to Ponder

36.6) How does knowing why God created us help us to understand our purpose?

36.7) How would you define God's main purpose for mankind, and for you personally?

His Plan and Purpose

And we know that God causes all things to work together for good to those who love God, to those who are called according to His purpose. For those whom He foreknew, He also predestined to become conformed to the image of His Son, so that He would be the firstborn among many brethren; http://biblehub.com/romans/8-30.htm*and these whom He predestined, He also called; and these whom He called, He also justified; and these whom He justified, He also glorified. What then shall we say to these things? If God is for us, who is against us? (Romans 8:28 – 31)*

God orchestrates all history for the benefit of those who are His. He knew our beginnings, our choices, and our ending before we ever were. Believers have a promise that He will redeem every moment of our life, forming it into good for us and others whom He has called.

➢ **Our purpose is to do His will.** You are predestined, meaning God planned you for this exact moment of time, so He could save all who would be saved. He plans to prosper each one of us, giving us a future and hope. The first and most important of those plans is to **draw us into proper relationship with Him** and transform us into His likeness.

➢ **Our purpose is love.** To be created in "God's likeness" means we shared God's attributes. It makes sense, then, that to restore our Christlikeness, we must be a people who love. Scripture states that we know followers of Jesus by their love for one another.

Your Life Has Purpose

God also has a specific plan and purpose for your life as an individual. Although God does require you to lay down your sin nature, he does not require you to give up who you are; **He made you unique to fulfill his purpose.** He equips each person with talents and gifts, whether we believe in Jesus or have any relationship at all with God.

We choose how we use our gifts. Those in the world who lack a relationship with Jesus often use their gifts and talents to prosper their own lives and fulfill the desires of their flesh. Those who live by the Spirit will take all that they are—their talents, gifts, and desires—and wrap them around the Lord to use for His glory and Kingdom purposes.

> You may find that God's mission is not the same as what you envisioned for your life. **Be assured**, however, that **His mission for you will fill you with joy**. You will experience satisfaction and fulfillment when you walk in His ways!

Consider ranks in the Army: a private has the least authority, and a general has the most authority. No other rank answers to the private, except when the general gives the private a mission. The private then carries the same authority as the general regarding that mission. **All** other ranks submit to him. **God is your general.** Everything submits to His authority, and when you are fulfilling His mission, you operate with His authority.

When we allow God to move **through** our gifts and talents, **we succeed**. God gives us gifts to help us **achieve the calling and purpose He has** for us. When we use our God-given abilities to carry out **His** plans, we cannot fail, because we have the power and authority of the Almighty God behind us.

> "If you live outside the will of God, if you act against it, then you will live and act with the authority of a private, which is to have no authority. But if you live inside the will of God, if you follow the directives of God, if you carry out His assignment, if you set your course on fulfilling His mission, then you will live in the authority of God. Then every rank in this universe must yield to your steps, every door must unlock, and every gate must open. So, make it your aim to live your life wholly in the will of God. Find your mission and fulfill it. … And you will walk in the power and authority of the Almighty."
>
> Jonathan Cahn, *The Book of Mysteries* (2016), "The Private and the General", p.133

Questions to Ponder

36.8) What do you think success in God's Kingdom looks like?

36.9) How does this differ from what the world sees as success?

36.10) What are your plans, your goals, dreams, and desires for the future? Seek the Lord about your purpose.

36.11) Can you imagine God prospering you in these pursuits? How?

36.12) Proverbs 19:21 says, "Many are the plans in the mind of a man, but it is the purpose of the LORD that will stand." What does this passage mean to you? Explain.

36.13) Are you okay with God's plans for your life, even if they differ from what you think you want? How will following His plans affect you?

Chapter Fourteen

Loving Who You
Are in Christ

Lesson 37 — Defining Love

How Important Is Love?

Love is everything. Without love we are nothing. We are able to love as a result of receiving God's love. We respond to His love and express our love for God by keeping His commandments. God's commandments are to love Him and to love others as ourselves. To overflow love into another, we must receive God's love. If our love for ourselves does not come from God, our attempts to love others will arise from a selfish need to fill an empty place in our heart. The more we love ourselves as God wants us to, the more we can love others as ourselves.

And if I have prophetic powers, and understand all mysteries and all knowledge, and if I have all faith, so as to remove mountains, <u>but have not love, I am nothing</u>. (1 Corinthians 13:2)

We love because he first loved us. (1 John 4:19)

➤ How do we love God? Jesus said the way we love Him is by keeping His commandments.

If you love me, <u>you will keep my commandments</u>. (John 14: 15)

Whoever has my commandments and keeps them, he it is who loves me. And he who loves me will be loved by my Father, and I will love him and manifest myself to him. (John 14:21)

➤ All God's commandments derive from these two: Love God and love others as yourself.

"Teacher, which is the great commandment in the Law?" And he said to him, "<u>You shall love the Lord your God</u> with all your heart and with all your soul and with all your mind. This is the great and first commandment. And a second is like it: <u>You shall love your neighbor as yourself</u>. On these two commandments depend all the Law and the Prophets. (Matthew 22:36 – 40)

➤ We are to love God, but to love God we must obey His commandment to love others.

Anyone who does not love does not know God, because God is love. (1 John 4:8)

If anyone says, "I love God," and hates his brother, he is a liar; for he who does not love his brother whom he has seen cannot love God whom he has not seen. (1 John 4:20)

Jesus commands us to love our neighbor (others) **as we love ourselves**. The more we love ourselves, the better we love others, and the more our love for God shows. The question then becomes, **"What does it mean to love yourself?"**

144

Loving Myself vs. Humility

You may wonder how you can have humility and love yourself. **Humility is not thinking less of yourself, it is thinking more of God.** It is building up another's qualities, not bragging about your own. It is esteeming others, giving them recognition before taking the glory for yourself. **Humility is not putting yourself down or treating yourself poorly.**

To gain more clarity about this, let us define what humility is and is not.

Humility is not:

- Thinking you are bad

- Seeing yourself as less valuable or worthy than another person

- Feeling or acting as if you do not matter

- Feeling or acting as if you are not good enough

The previous list describes, not humility, but humiliation. Humiliation actually masks pride. When we act in humiliation, we want others to feed our pride in order to combat our insecurity. People who live in humiliation often behave pridefully, as if they are secure and confident, but they do this to hide their insecurity.

Humility is:

- Seeing yourself honestly, **not as more or less** than you are

- Knowing that without God you can do nothing, but with God you can do all things

- Esteeming others over yourself **without** regarding them as having greater worth

- Feeling or acting as if you do not matter

- Feeling or acting as if you are not good enough

- Giving others respect, admiration, and honor **before** accepting it for yourself

- Knowing that you have value that comes, **not from yourself, but from God**

- Living a life led by the Lord and **dying to your own will**

Humility is the first step in loving yourself because humility is where God changes your heart. Here is a saying to remember when you are struggling in your relationship with God: **Pride prevents progress**. For God to change your life, you must have the attitude that He knows better than you.

> ### Questions to Ponder
>
> 37.1) Do you act in humiliation or in humility?
>
> 37.2) How has your pride prevented God from making progress with you in your journey?
>
> 37.3) When looking at yourself, do you like or dislike what you see?
>
> 37.4) Can you say that you love yourself? Describe what you feel about yourself.

We tend to act from self-preservation when we believe we are undeserving of love, have a poor self-image, or carry deep shame. **This makes it impossible to show selfless love** to others. When strongholds like fear or anger dictate our thinking, they filter how we see others. **We often assume people think and act the same way we would in any given situation.** When we are stuck in shame and wrong thoughts about ourselves, we are more likely to misjudge others' motives as well. We struggle to love others properly because we "love" them **out of our own need** for love instead of a desire to give of ourselves to them.

> Our ability to love our neighbor is dependent on how we value ourselves.
> With a godly view of ourselves, we are able to give and receive God's kind of love!

Love Defined

People tend to abuse the word *love*. People can also abuse others in the name of love, or use "love" to manipulate others for their own selfish ends. When we have difficulty trusting in other people's love, we will struggle to trust God's love. We may see God as either a harsh judge or uninvolved. However, Scripture says God is **love**. If we cannot understand God's love, we will never have a correct perception of God.

Everybody agrees love is good, but we do not agree on what love is. **It is impossible to accept or display a love we do not understand.** Today, many people equate love with gushy emotions, selfish desires, or sexual intimacy. I love my friend. I love pizza. I love my first crush … and then next year, I love another. We have deeper forms of love also, such as the love for our children, spouse, parents, and God. These experiences are all different, yet we use the same word, love, to describe them all. Love has become very confusing.

The two Hebrew words used in the Bible to express love are *ahava* and *chesed*, and these words give a clearer understanding of God's love. ***Ahava* and *chesed* display attributes of God.** The writers of the New Testament Greek used the word ***agape*** to attempt to capture the meaning of these two Hebrew words.

CHESED: This word can express love from God to people, or between people.
- o Translations describe *chesed* as **loving-kindness, mercy, steadfast love, compassion, loyalty, goodness, great kindness, favor, and loyalty.** It is an **unfailing, everlasting, steadfast, and loyal love**, an **eternal faithfulness** or **devotion**.

- o *Chesed* is **unselfish love**, and it is proven in actions performed **with no thought of "what's in it for me?"** The expression of this kind of love is **not dependent on your mood or what you feel.**

- o *Chesed* is **a love that surpasses your own hurts.** It overcomes the harm people do through their words, their sin, and their betrayal. *Chesed*'s **compassion motivates** us to extend grace, mercy, and forgiveness.

- o *Chesed* is more than charity *(tzedakah)*. It is an **excess or overflowing** of kindness, going beyond what is required or expected. *Chesed* **produces** abundant, extravagant giving and acts of charity, mercy, and kindness toward someone in a greater measure than they deserve**.**
   The Pharisees performed acts of charity *(tzedakah)*; Jesus expected love *(chesed)*.

AHAVA: This word represents our love toward God. It is selfless, not dependent upon what He does for us. We express this love through action, and therefore it is **a choice**.

- o *Ahava* is both a noun and a verb representing both the actions of love and the feeling of love. It represents a feeling **because** of an action, not an action as the **result** of a feeling.

- o The root word *ahav* means **to give**. Therefore, this love **is not something that happens to you**, but something that **comes from you**. Your act of giving generates *ahava*, regardless of whether the giving is of your affection, time, or resources.

- o *Avaha* should be **the intent** behind our thoughts, words, and actions, and our motivation for obedience in response to Jesus' command: "If you love Me, you will keep My commandments" (John 14:15).

AGAPE: This is the most used and important word for love found in the New Testament.

- o It is the closest word in the Greek to express the Hebrew concept of selfless love.

- o This love relates to what God prefers, to his ways, as "God is love" (1 Jn 4:8,16), and therefore it **relates to righteousness**. The greatest act of love was Jesus giving His life to cover the sins of mankind and make us righteous in His sight!

These words for love create a picture of the love Jesus calls us to have for God, our neighbors, and ourselves. **In none of these words do we find the connotation of a feeling creating love.** We can love others without feeling it. It is often after we exhibit love that we experience the resulting emotion. This is easier to understand when we think about loving other people or God, but **more difficult when we think about loving ourselves**.

> **⓵ QUICK FACT**
>
> Many people are familiar with the Greek word *agape* used to describe love in the New Testament, but did you know there are two other Greek words occasionally used to express love?
>
> *Storge* **describes love for family, and** *phileo* **describes the love you would have for a close friend.** *Phileo* is affection based in feelings, or it can be a sentiment toward an object. *(I love pizza.)*
>
> **These words do not speak to a godly or sacrificial love.**

Questions to Ponder

37.5) What are the attributes of a biblical love?

37.6) How has your understanding of the nature and expression of love changed after reading this lesson?

37.7) What attributes of God can you identify as love?

37.8) What parts of Scripture do you find difficult to accept as God's love?

37.9) For each thing you mentioned in answering the previous question, describe how each could be an act or expression of God's love.

37.10) Describe how you can love yourself without "feeling it".

Why Righteousness?

Is it love to enable someone to continue in destructive sin? Of course not! **Love corrects and protects.** It is that very question that leads us to know that **every** attribute of God is love. His justice, authority (law), and judgment are love as much as his grace and mercy are love. It can be easier to accept God's discipline for someone who hurt you than to accept His discipline for yourself. The Lord compares his reproof to a father disciplining His son. While it is uncomfortable, He intends it to help us mature.

> *My son, do not despise the LORD's discipline or be weary of his reproof, for the LORD reproves him whom he loves, as a father the son in whom he delights.*
> *(Proverbs 3:11 – 12)*

> *Have you forgotten the exhortation that addresses you as sons? My son, do not regard lightly the discipline of the Lord nor be weary when reproved by him. For the Lord disciplines the one he loves and chastises every son whom he receives. It is for discipline that you have to endure. God is treating you as sons. For what son is there whom his father does not discipline? If you are left without discipline, in which all have participated, then you are illegitimate children and not sons.*
> *(Hebrews 12:5 – 7)*

A Heavenly Father's Love

God designed the family to teach us about Himself and about love. In a fallen world, however, our families are flawed, sometimes with significant dysfunction. Since no one has a perfect family, **we must not attribute their flaws and failures to God**. His Word can make up where families fall short. God is the perfect father, teaching and helping us to grow, but **He is not abusive or cruel**. He never leaves us to fight our battles alone, but stands by our side. His discipline is for our welfare and not to harm us. **He convicts us of our sin, like a good father** who instructs his son about right and wrong, **and He is our safety net**, so the consequences of our sins do not destroy us.

> *"Do not fear, O Jacob My servant," says the LORD, "For I am with you; For I will make a complete end of all the nations to which I have driven you, but I will not make a complete end of you. I will rightly correct you, for I will not leave you wholly unpunished." (Jeremiah 46:28)*

God's discipline is not punishment for the sake of punishment. Discipline may include a natural consequence, but it is designed to teach us and help us grow into wholeness and perfection, preparing us for eternity. God's discipline is always out of love and always for our benefit.

> *Count it all joy, my brothers, when you meet trials of various kinds, for you know that the testing of your faith produces steadfastness. And let steadfastness have its full effect, that you may be perfect and complete, lacking in nothing.*
> *(James 1:2 – 4)*

Questions to Ponder

37.11) Describe God as a father.

37.12) Describe the love you received from your parents as a child. How was their love a good representation of God's love?

37.13) In what ways was the parenting you received as a child a poor representation of God's love?

37.14) How is your love for your spouse teaching you about a loving relationship with Christ as His bride? *(If you are not married, how can you imagine love for a spouse teaching you about this relationship with Christ?)*

37.15) How can your marriage *(or future marriage)* be a bad example of relationship with Christ?

Lesson 38 — Addressing Shame

Questions to Ponder

38.1) Do you *feel* like you love yourself?

38.2) How do you treat yourself with love?

38.3) Think about the definitions of love in the previous lesson. Based on these definitions, how can you love yourself better?

Are You Bad?

Surely I was brought forth in iniquity; I was sinful when my mother conceived me. (Psalm 51:5)

Among whom we all once lived in the passions of our flesh, carrying out the desires of the body and the mind, and were by nature children of wrath, like the rest of mankind.
(Ephesians 2:3)

Do you ever feel confused when you try to think of yourself as righteous, justified, or a saint? Would you call yourself "good"? How do you reconcile the idea that you are righteous when you know your sinful thoughts and ways? If you are always confident in your righteousness, you are in the minority. Maybe you compare yourself to "better" Christians, wear a Christian mask, or fall short of your expectations. When you examine your heart and see the sin and wickedness within, it may be difficult to "feel" righteous, **yet Scripture says our faith is our righteousness and our justification is by the sacrifice of Jesus**.

Defining Good and Bad

God did not design good to exist apart from Him. He is good, and apart from Him nothing can be good. **Therefore, evil is what exists in the absence of God, and sin is the force which perpetuates evil.** The evil, hardship, and destructive force of decay and death were **not** God's design for this world. These things resulted from sin entering the world. The same pattern that ensnared Eve in the garden continues today, as shown in the book of James. No one is exempt from sin.

But each person is tempted when he is lured and enticed by his own desire. Then desire when it has conceived gives birth to sin, and sin when it is fully grown brings forth death.
(James 1:14 – 15)

Eve had distorted thoughts when the enemy **tempted her** to disobey God. Her **desire for wisdom enticed** her, and then the desire **gave birth to her plan of action**: eating the fruit. The sin committed **brought forth death**, or separation from God. Mankind lost their divine nature, exchanging it for an "evil nature"—our sin nature.

God knitted each of us together in the womb as a perfect creation, yet we are tainted at conception by sin's power. God did not create wicked people. He created people who became wicked because they have a corrupting sin nature. **Only God can change it.**

There is good news, though: **God knew this would happen and developed a backup plan**, even before laying the foundations of the earth. Jesus agreed to pay the penalty for our sin with His own blood, thus removing the separation of man from God, bringing life, and allowing us to regain fellowship with God. We become clean from our sin; our divine nature restored. As we head into our eternal existence, we will receive a new, incorruptible body, unaffected by the power of sin.

What does this mean to you? By accepting Christ as your Lord and Savior, you gave God permission to **change your nature**. In Christ, you must no longer carry the label of bad, the label of shame. You are a **redeemed saint** living in an evil world with a **nature prone to sin**. You will never be perfect while living on this earth, but your life in Christ will show fruit of **His likeness**. We have a promise that one day we will be perfect and complete, lacking in nothing, if we can persevere. **Becoming Christlike is a life-long process.**

> ## Questions to Ponder
>
> 38.4) In what areas of your life do you feel inadequate?
>
> 38.5) How do you handle your mistakes?
>
> 38.6) In what ways do you allow past failures and mistakes to define you?
>
> 38.7) How should your thoughts regarding your sin and shame change?

Labels

From our earliest moments we want to define things. Born with curiosity about our world and ourselves, we look to others to understand our place. We begin life mimicking behaviors and actions we see, attempting to discover our limits and our identity.

This process covers us with labels. As our vocabulary grows, the label game begins. Every experience, mistake, assumption, and influence adds a label. We strive to be special and unique, to excel, and to stand out because we want to define our labels. These labels become our identity.

Identity labels

We project the identity labels we want others to see in us—labels like powerful, secure, and creative. These **identity labels are our "walls."** We cover ourselves in these walls to give us a sense of self-worth and value. We seek people with similar walls to find belonging. Identity labels define how our mind perceives the person we **should be**.

As we go through life, **people attempt to modify our labels with their own**. (You are pretty, ugly, the love of my life, a brat ...) The negative labels people and our experiences place on us become shame in our hearts. Shame creates more shame as our own minds betray us, reinforcing this distorted picture of ourselves.

Shame Labels

The Insults and condemnation other people claim for us produce shame labels. These labels may also come from expectations others want us to meet, or from praise and flattery for an image we cannot maintain. Shame labels shape how our mind perceives the person **we are**. We bury shame labels deep beneath our walls (our identity labels) to keep them hidden.

The way others treat us and their words are a powerful influence guiding our perception of our worth. People's words and our circumstances continually reinforce this skewed perception. The enemy takes advantage, whispering lies that we are not enough: not good enough, not smart enough, not attractive enough, not successful enough. We then end up comparing ourselves to others or to some unachievable expectations we decide we must meet.

Our insecurities drive us to be better and better, but we always seem to fall short of our "enoughs." This reinforces the labels others have given us. We then make a choice to either accept those labels or combat them with our own. **Yet the truth is that none of these labels define us.** The only accurate labels are the ones given to us by the Lord, and therefore, believing the label lies of ourselves and others, leads to shame.

What is shame? We all make mistakes and have varying degrees of guilt. We do wrong, apologize, try to make it right, and then move on. However, sometimes our mistakes reinforce negative beliefs we have about ourselves. **We exchange the guilt of *doing* something bad for a deep-seated belief that we *are* something bad.** This is the shame that keeps us defeated.

Words influence how we understand our identity, but our labels do not define us. **They are just a sticker on the outside of the package with a misleading ingredients list**, giving us a false view of our worth. If we believe our labels, we will become either pumped up in pride, or waste away in shame and feelings of worthlessness.

Questions to Ponder

38.8) **What words or actions of your parents or caregivers when you were a child influence your thoughts or reactions now?**

38.9) **What words or events from your early childhood sent you positive messages?**

38.10) **What words or events from your early childhood reinforced your shame?**

38.11) **Consider your teen and adult years. How have events and words affected your internal belief about your worth?**

38.12) **List the identity labels that define you.**

38.13) **List the shame labels that define you.**

38.14) **Reflect again about the labels that define you. Do you see anything new or recent?**

38.15) **What experience caused each shame or identity label you listed?**

38.16) **Looking back on the labels you have believed throughout your life, how have your shame and identity labels influenced your responses?**

You are *not* what you do.
You are *not* your past, your failures, or your mistakes.
Only the Lord defines your identity.

Lesson 39 — Your Path Defines You

How Do You *Know* Who You Are Beneath Your Masks and Labels?

All people are:

Created for relationship with God

Created for love and to love

Created for righteousness

People have a choice:

Choose to accept and become the person they were created to become

Choose to pursue self and cling to their sin nature

The person we desire to become shows our heart, the genuine person existing deep in our soul. We may not like our actions, but **our actions do not define us; our path defines us.**

Our Path Defines Us

If we choose to **satisfy our sin nature**, rejecting God's ways, then we travel on **a path of destruction, and the enemy gets to define our identity**. If we choose **God's path** and pursue righteousness, then **He defines our identity**.

For example, a man whose deepest desire of his heart is to become rich or powerful might use any method to achieve that desire. He may steal, cheat, manipulate, or use people to reach his goals, feeling justified in doing so. **His desires and motives** are for self and reveal who he truly is and the path of life he has chosen.

Another man may desire wealth, but the deepest desire of his heart is to help people and invest into the lives of others. His desire for riches is for investment into his community. He strives for that success, but his heart's desire is to be someone who loves people. His desires and motives also show his true identity and a path after the heart of God.

Nearly everyone desires success, but not everyone defines success the same way. Success to some looks like the world: prosperity, notoriety, position, power. For others it looks like a happy family, raising successful kids, bringing people to know Jesus, or serving and investing in the lives of others. How you define success is another important key to defining who you are. **It is not the desire, but the motive in your heart fueling the desire which reveals your path.** When your motives line up with God's will, you can be assured you are on His path.

Questions to Ponder

39.1) Imagine what the perfect person would be like? Describe details of his or her character, personality, and abilities. (Your perfect person would be one you can admire, respect, and want to be like—someone you would become if it were possible. Note: this is hypothetical. No one is perfect.)

39.2) Is the person you described worthy of your love? Is it someone you want to become?

39.3) Do you think you can become like this person? Why or why not?

39.4) Define the deepest desires of your heart regarding the character and identity you desire for yourself. Be honest.

39.5) How do you define success for your life?

39.6) Narrow your definition of a successful life to one achievement that gives your life value and meaning.

39.7) Describe the path in life that you have chosen.

Good News

Your picture of a perfect person reflects the person you desire to become. **Your perfect person reflects the values of your heart!** This person is inside you, waiting to come out.

Sometimes our beliefs of what makes someone "good" are based on other people's perceptions of the right way to be in life. Parents, teachers, role models, and friends have instilled in us some of their beliefs.

If your perfect person does not line up with the deep desires of your heart, you may be listening to a voice that is not your own. For example, if your dad raised you to never show weakness, your perfect person may have characteristics of safety and strength, never showing emotion or pain. However, when you defined your deepest desires, you may have included empathy for others. You cannot have empathy for someone without emotions. The person in this example is double minded in this area. He would need to examine what he really feels and believes apart from what others have told him or modeled for him. Before you can determine who you really are as a person, or if your beliefs are right or wrong, you must sort through and discover **what you think for yourself**.

**The character and personality of your perfect person,
how you define success, and the spiritual path you choose define you.**
In Christ, this is the person God created you to be, and this is a person you can love. Strive with the Lord to become that person!

Questions to Ponder

39.8)   If your perfect person does not match up to the deepest desires of your heart, how are they different?

39.9)   Do you have some ways of thinking that are not your genuine beliefs, but the beliefs of another? What are they?

Questions to Ponder

39.10) Examine your answers to all the questions from this lesson. Use the characteristics of your perfect person, your definition of success, and the path you have chosen for life to write what life would look like as your perfect person.

39.11) Read your answer to the previous question. This description describes who your heart says you are. What does this say about your identity, potential, and purpose?

Find three people whose opinion matters most to you and have each one list everything they like about you, especially referring to your character. Each person should seal their lists in an envelope. Do not look at what they wrote ... yet.

Chapter Fifteen

Identifying &
Removing Lies

Lesson 40 — Who You Are in Christ

In Christ, we have a new identity. As we discovered in the last lesson, we are transforming into a new creation. So, what is this new identity? Where does our worth come from? You have identified your walls (identity labels) and your shame (lies you believe about yourself); now it is **time to reveal your real label.**

The Lord gives you a seal, which is your genuine label. The Holy Spirit confirms your seal, bearing witness with your own spirit that you belong to Him. Then He begins transforming you into the righteous new creation promised by your faith in Christ.

And it is God who <u>establishes us</u> with you in Christ, and has <u>anointed us</u>, and who has also <u>put his seal on us</u> and given us <u>his Spirit</u> in our hearts <u>as a guarantee</u>. (2 Corinthians 1:21 – 22)

The following are just a few of the scriptures that describe our identity in Christ:

- *"Do you not know you are <u>God's temple</u> and that God's Spirit dwells in you?" (1 Corinthians 3:16)*

- *"No longer do I call you servants, for the servant does not know what his master is doing; but <u>I have called you friends</u>." (John 15:15)*

- *"But to all who did receive him ... he gave the right to become <u>children of God</u>." (John 1:12)*

- *"But you are a <u>chosen race, a royal priesthood, a holy nation, a people for his own possession</u>, that you may proclaim the excellencies of him who called you out of darkness into his marvelous light." (1 Peter 2:9)*

- *"Therefore, if anyone is in Christ, he is <u>a new creation</u>." (2 Corinthians 5:17)*

In Christ we are secure, sealed, protected, and sustained
despite our circumstances or past sins.

How does God see you? Scripture tells us everyone has sinned and fallen short of the Glory of God. Why would God, the creator of heaven and earth, want to be your friend? How does that happen?

God hates sin because it separates us from Him. He is holy and righteous, and He cannot be with evil. How can God look at us, people who do evil, and claim we are righteous? In the Old Testament, He even called David, an adulterer and murderer, a man after His own heart. How can this be?

God sees our final product. He is the Alpha and Omega, the beginning and the end. He sees the past, future, and all points in between. We go through life as if traveling a straight line in front of us, only seeing one step ahead and everything behind us. God, however, sees life from a full perspective of history. He has a bird's-eye view of our lives. He knows the person He created us to be and the person we will become. **Therefore, we look at ourselves and see one thing, but God looks at us and sees something completely different!**

157

The Lord fixes His eyes on who we are becoming, not who we are now.

We see ourselves:	He sees us:
In turmoil	Peaceful
Broken	Healed
Rejected	Chosen
Without a voice	God's ambassador
Guilty and condemned	Righteous and justified
Fearful	Faithful
Trapped	Free
A mistake	Ordained with purpose
A failure/loser	Successful/victorious
Worthless	Valuable
Weak	Strong
No future	With a future and hope
Ugly/disabled/diseased	Fearfully and wonderfully made

We Are a Work in Progress

What does the process of creating a prized sculpture look like? The sculpture starts out as nothing more than a lump of clay. The sculptor begins shaping the clay. You can only catch a hint of what he is creating. As it nears completion the clay looks more like the finished product, but it is still flawed. You cannot see its flawless beauty until the sculptor completes his work. Likewise, we are incomplete, still in the molding process, with the potential to become glorious!

Imagine if the lump of clay spoke and had free will. What if it said, "No, I am ugly, I am only clay?" What if the clay became so set on its flawed appearance that it refused to allow the sculptor to work? It would never transform. It would forever remain an ugly lump of clay.

If you created a masterpiece, would you throw your work away? Would that masterpiece have value? You are God's masterpiece, a lump of clay in your maker's hands. With every work God does in your heart, you are becoming closer to the image of perfection that God promises for you, a beautiful sculpture in His hands, in the likeness of your creator. He gives another promise, too: He will complete the work He began in you! Focus on the person you are becoming and leave the shame of the past in the past.

And I am sure of this, that he who began a good work in you will bring
it to completion at the day of Jesus Christ. (Philippians 1:6)

Discerning Truth and Deception

This world disguises bad as good and good as bad. If Satan walked up to you looking evil, you would reject him. Instead, **he disguises his lies as truth**, feeding off your self-doubt and insecurity. His lies are reinforced by the harsh words and actions of others and validated as you make comparisons and try to measure up to false standards. You lie to your soul with each thought that screams you are not good enough. Who is good enough?

But when they measure themselves by one another and compare
themselves with one another, they are without understanding.
(2 Corinthians 10:12)

Sometimes the deception you believe **is not lies masked in a disguise of truth, but a truth hidden by a lie**. Like a forest in the winter, every tree appears dead. The teeming life of the forest is hidden away, waiting for the spring. Walking in the woods on a winter day, the appearance of death is stark. For a person unfamiliar with the seasons, it may seem impossible to believe life exists in this barren place.

This illusion of death is necessary for life to flourish in a winter forest. The snow keeps the winter plants insulated and provides moisture for the harsh conditions. Frigid temperatures limit pests that would damage fragile plants and bacteria that cause disease. Trees and plants lie dormant and rest from growing. Like a deep sleep, this rest builds the plants' energy, enabling fresh growth and strengthening the plant to produce more seeds and fruit. **The lie of death hides the reality of life.**

Likewise, your shame is a lie with the appearance of death, making you believe you are incapable, unworthy, a failure, with no hope for success or life. It is a lie so loud, supported by so much false evidence, that you do not question it. Why would you seek another answer? If you are convinced a lie is truth, your thoughts and actions will defend the belief. Abundant life may seem impossible, but if you overcome the lie of your winter, you will find purpose and life.

Knowing God's truth **unravels lies** and **removes their power**. You must keep your mind stayed on His Word and the truth of who you are in Christ. **To overcome your labels, you must have different thoughts.** You must **choose** to consider yourself as God sees you.

When you perceive yourself as not____ enough (good enough, smart enough, thin enough, successful enough, etc.), remember God is not finished yet. **You are enough for God.** When you seem to fail, remember God makes you victorious. Mistakes do not equal failure. When you are unable, know it is God who makes you able. When you feel broken, remember that you are being healed. When you are scared, remember you are protected. **Surrender your old, broken self to the Lord and let Him redefine you!**

It is hard to love yourself
when you are deceived about who you are.

Take these five steps to stop the lies:

1. **Give up** your mess to God.

2. **Identify** the truth—the report of the Lord.

3. **Remind** yourself of that truth.

4. **Recognize** the report the enemy speaks to you.

5. **Stop** believing the lies!

<u>Questions to Ponder</u>

40.1) Who is good enough?

40.2) How have you let your mistakes define you? Do you trust that what the Lord says defines you? Why or why not?

40.3) In what ways do you recognize the Lord working in your heart to redefine some labels you have been believing?

40.4) How do you struggle to see the Lord working to change you? What is stopping that change?

40.5) What must you overcome to surrender to these changes?

40.6) List everything you like about yourself, especially regarding your character.

Open the lists you had others make about you in the homework from the last lesson.

40.7) What are the similarities to your lists?

40.8) Which of their answers are not on your list?

40.9) Do their answers surprise you? Why or why not?

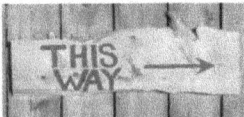

Ask your coach for more information about who you are in Christ

Introduction to Book Four

Your Journey Home — The Future

You have learned many things through this journey: how to love yourself, identify the enemy's lies, trust God in your hurt, and turn to Him when you mess up. You walk through life with the Lord by your side. Remember how far you have come!

As you begin this book, you might be experiencing a mixture of emotions. You may feel confident in your progress and ready for this journey to end, or you may be concerned about repeating past mistakes and questioning your ability to discern truth from lies. This book will help you hone the skills needed to maintain your victory, stay confident, and prevent a relapse into old thinking.

The enemy is always in your ear, wanting you to fail, but you know a secret: He loses! God turns his plans upside down. All the enemy meant for your destruction becomes your blessing. You will not fear falling when you remain diligent and keep your eyes on your source.

The close of one journey begins another. Your relationship with the Lord grows deeper as your life begins to flow forth from His. The lessons in this book will teach you to fight spiritual enemies, have strong relationships, handle conflict, and step forward.

In This Book

Your Journey Home
You have a hidden enemy trying to sabotage your future. Conquer your flesh by making the Lord your only stronghold.

Choosing Healthy Relationships
Learn about healthy and toxic relationships, and about setting boundaries. You will also learn how to identify detrimental behaviors in yourself and others.

Conflict Resolution
An in-depth look at resolving conflicts and establishing effective communication.

Moving Forward
Learn to live *from* God instead of *for* Him. Establish useful habits to protect your focus from slipping. Write your story and discover ways to serve with *Rebuilt*.

Chapter Sixteen

Your Journey Home

Lesson 41 — Your Journey Home

How do you feel knowing your time with *Rebuilt* is coming to an end? It is the close of one season in a lifelong quest. Your growth does not cease when you complete the last page of this book. The deep-rooted sin and strongholds interwoven in your heart are difficult to pull out. You may notice you are continuing to be tested in old strongholds and problematic thinking patterns, or you may discover new ones. This is the Lord's way to **fortify your freedom** and **strengthen your faith** in Him. The tools you have learned have set you on the right course to weather future challenges and make the Lord your only stronghold.

The LORD is my light and my salvation; whom shall I fear?
The LORD is the stronghold of my life; of whom shall I be afraid? (Psalm 27:1)

The Lord is a stronghold for the oppressed a stronghold in times of trouble. And those who know your name put their trust in you, for you, O Lord, have not forsaken those who seek you. (Psalm 9:9 – 10)

Process of Progress

Healing the hurts in your heart is like cleaning out a physical wound. Slapping a bandage over a serious wound without giving it proper care and treatment traps all the yuck inside, allowing infection to fester and spread to the rest of the body. To properly care for a wound, you must cleanse it thoroughly. You must debride the wound to prevent any infection from remaining. The deeper the wound, the deeper you must go to clear it out.

In the past you used many things, perhaps even Jesus, as a Band-Aid® to cover emotional and spiritual wounds without dealing with the root or cause of the injury. Just as with physical injuries, the longer you allow an emotional hurt to fester, the more digging is required to remove the corruption it caused.

By this point, you have **pulled off your emotional bandage, cut away the damage, and cleared the festering infection underneath**. You no longer cover up your wounds, pretend they do not exist, or believe they can improve on their own. But even with proper treatment, deep emotional trauma takes time to heal. You may experience complete freedom in some areas while infection is still being purged in others. The process peels back layer after layer until the Lord reveals every hidden poison in your heart.

This book will serve as an aid to strengthen and prepare you for the continuing journey ahead. The principles presented here are meant to help you **prevent relapse** and **continue the healing process**. You will further your relationship with God, develop healthy relationships, establish reasonable boundaries, and foster better communication.

Where Are You?

You made considerable progress on this journey. Before continuing, take a moment to assess your growth. This will prepare you to deal with future struggles and give you confidence in your successes. **For each question that follows, state how much you thought or believed the idea before you started this journey, and how much you believe the idea now. Is there a large change? Are there areas where you would like to see more change?**

166

<u>Questions to Ponder</u>

Provide two answers for each question below, one for before you started this journey and one for where you are now. State your answers as either percentages, or on a scale of 1 to 10, with 1 being not at all and 10 being the maximum amount.

41.1)   How well did/do you learn from your failures?

41.2)   How often did/are you choosing change (doing and thinking differently)?

41.3)   How much were/are you living for God?

41.4)   How much were/are you living to survive?

41.5)   How much did/do you trust God's Word is true *for you*?

41.6)   How secure were/are you in your relationship with God?

41.7)   How much trust did/do you give God?

41.8)   How often did/do you hear God's voice?

41.9)   Were/Are you bandaging your wounds or facing them?

41.10) How much did/do you believe that God invests in you? Explain.

Consider your responses to the previous questions when answering the following.

41.11) In what ways do you trust God, both now and before your journey began?

41.12) In what areas do you recognize the most change since beginning *Rebuilt*?

41.13) In which areas do you note the most change?

41.14) In which areas do you note the least change?

41.15) Where would you prefer to see more change or improvement?

Where Are You Headed?

Head for the finish line! This life is a race to eternity, a training ground for our future. The prize? A crown, a kingdom, an eternal existence with no pain or tears. Keep your eyes on the prize. God's Word says not to grow weary of doing good. Do not give up! Stand firm and confident!

Do you not know that in a race all the runners run, but only one receives the prize? So run that you may obtain it. Every athlete exercises self-control in all things. They do it to receive a perishable wreath, but we imperishable. (1 Corinthians 9:24 – 25)

I have fought the good fight, I have finished the race, I have kept the faith. (2 Timothy 4:7)

And I am sure of this, that he who began a good work in you will bring it to completion at the day of Jesus Christ. (Philippians 1:6)

And let us not grow weary of doing good, for in due season we will reap, if we do not give up. (Galatians 6:9)

<u>Questions to Ponder</u>

41.16) How have your priorities changed? Define your priorities for the future.

41.17) How do you see your life unfolding differently after *Rebuilt*?

41.18) How does this differ from what you expected for your life before you began *Rebuilt*?

Lesson 42 — A Surprising Enemy

You have a spiritual enemy who hates you, especially because of your relationship with the Lord. He will do anything to make you ineffective in God's Kingdom. To combat this enemy, you must first understand him. **His main stomping ground is the undisciplined mind.** He speaks lies and tempts us, **but it is our choices, not Satan, that make us sin**.

Your thoughts and desires birth sin. Satan inhabits your sin, using it as a doorway into your life. Satan capitalizes on your fearful or wrong thinking to conceive desires, tempting you to act on sinful thoughts (i.e., any thought which goes against the Word of God). He uses the sin in you to steal, kill, and destroy.

> *But each person is tempted when he is <u>lured and enticed by his own desire</u>. Then desire when it has conceived gives birth to sin, and sin when it is fully grown brings forth death.*
> *(James 1:14 – 15)*

Sin is the **power** behind your **enemy**, but **we have free will.** When we **choose life and live**, the Lord will take what Satan meant to destroy us and use it for our good.

> *I call heaven and earth to witness against you today, that I have set before you life and death, blessing and curse. Therefore choose life, that you and your offspring may live.*
> *(Deuteronomy 30:19)*

God's word tells us to have the mind of Christ because the mind is where our battle begins. Satan whispers lies in our ear, but with the mind of Christ, sin is dead in us and Satan's influence diminishes. When we have the Lord, we recognize that our greatest enemy is our own flesh.

> *Since therefore Christ suffered in the flesh, <u>arm yourselves with the same way of thinking</u>, for whoever has <u>suffered in the flesh has ceased from sin</u>, so as to live for the rest of the time in the flesh no longer for human passions but for the will of God. (1 Peter 4:1 – 2)*

Having the mind of Christ is not considering ourselves equal with God; rather, it is exalting God and emptying ourselves to be filled with His Spirit. We exchange our own ways, thoughts, and desires for God's ways, thoughts, and desires.

> *<u>Have this mind among yourselves, which is\ yours in Christ Jesus</u>, who, though he was in the form of God, did not count equality with God a thing to be grasped, but emptied himself, by taking the form of a servant, being born in the likeness of men. (Philippians 2:5 – 7)*

Jesus served as our example. He emptied himself, sacrificing his divine position to be born a man, and he was humbled, even to death on a cross. He subjected any desire of His flesh in obedience to the Father's will, and God exalted him for this. Jesus knew **humanity's greatest struggle** was trying to grasp equality with God—a goal we could never attain. Since the enemy tempted Eve with the words "you will be like God, knowing good and evil" (Genesis 3:5), we all fight against this same sin. We want to be **God over our own self, our own purpose, and our own thoughts**. When you realize you will never be God and empty yourself, **God will exalt you**.

Having a mind like Christ means our ways are acceptable to our righteous God. If Jesus were sitting next to you, would you watch that movie with Him? Would you listen to that music or play that game? Would you speak the way you speak to others? What about the thoughts in your mind? Would you speak those thoughts out loud to Jesus? Is your anger righteous?

A discipled mind is crucial to your continuing walk with the Lord!

Questions to Ponder

42.1) Consider your recent actions, thoughts, and words. Write both positive and negative examples of each.

42.2) In what situations were you negative?

42.3) When do the opinions of men guide you instead of the opinions of God?

Examine your answers above. For each item you mentioned:

42.4) In what ways did you have a mind like Christ?

42.5) In what ways are you trying to be God over your own life or other situations?

Patience Please, Your Flesh Is Fighting for Survival

For I do not understand my own actions. For I do not do what I want, but I do the very thing I hate. Now if I do what I do not want, I agree with the law, that it is good. So now it is no longer I who do it, but sin that dwells within me. For I know that nothing good dwells in me, that is, in my flesh. For I have the desire to do what is right, but not the ability to carry it out. For I do not do the good I want, but the evil I do not want is what I keep on doing. Now if I do what I do not want, it is no longer I who do it, but sin that dwells within me. (Romans 7:15 – 20)

Freedom comes as the Lord removes the root of the wrong thoughts that cause our sin. When we suffer in the flesh and overcome, **we cease sinning** in that area. The power of sin still works in areas of our life in which we continue acting in wrong, harmful ways. Have patience with your suffering flesh; it is dying to sin, and it wants to live. Remember, when your heart's desire is to do right, but you still do wrong, **your mistakes do not define you**. It is your sin nature.

The True Replacement Theology

The blood of Jesus makes us righteous. He paid the price to remove our sin from us. Why does it matter when we continue to sin if He forgives it?

If we say we have no sin, we deceive ourselves, and the truth is not in us. (1 John 1:8)

As Christians, we are being transformed into a bride without blemish, suitable to marry a king! We were **made righteous** by Jesus' sacrifice, and we are **being made holy**, set apart for the Lord. By following Christ, our lives reflect a transformation that serves as a witness of Him to the world. God promises to continue **taking us from one measure of glory to the next**.

And we all, with unveiled face, beholding the glory of the Lord, are being transformed into the same image from one degree of glory to another. For this comes from the Lord who is the Spirit. (2 Corinthians 3:18)

And I am sure of this, that he who began a good work in you will bring it to completion at the day of Jesus Christ. (Philippians 1:6)

The Replacement

If we are to become the new creation in Christ, **God must replace our sin nature with His nature** by a process of put-offs and put-ons, replacing our old ways with new. **Both natures cannot exist together.** Scripture shows this process through a vision of Joshua, the high priest.

Then he showed me Joshua the high priest standing before the angel of the LORD, and Satan standing at his right hand to accuse him. And the LORD said to Satan, "The LORD rebuke you, O Satan! The LORD who has chosen Jerusalem rebuke you! Is not this a brand plucked from the fire?" Now Joshua was standing before the angel, clothed with filthy garments. And the angel said to those who were standing before him, "Remove the filthy garments from him." And to him he said, "Behold, I have taken your iniquity away from you, and I will clothe you with pure vestments." And I said, "Let them put a clean turban on his head." So they put a clean turban on his head and clothed him with garments. And the angel of the LORD was standing by. (Zechariah 3:1 – 5)

This passage paints a symbolic picture of our transformation into a "new man." Satan and the Lord are arguing for Joshua. The Lord removes his filthy garments (the sin nature), replacing them with pure vestments (righteousness). **It is not enough to stop sinning. We must replace what we cast off with something new: Christ.**

In the New Testament, Paul teaches us what things we should put off or put on using the Greek word ***enduo***. It refers to putting on and taking off clothing. Paul is addressing both what must be removed from our lives, like filthy garments, and in what we should clothe ourselves.

Consider your routine when you get up in the morning to start your day as a picture of God's plan for redemption. First, you take off your dirty clothes. This is like when you realize you must turn away from your sin. Then you hop in the shower. This is like when begin to become spiritually clean by acknowledging the sacrifice of Jesus to pay the price of your sin. You are clean, but before you are free to go, you must get dressed.

After you bathe, you put on undergarments so your clothing fits properly. This is like putting on Christ and abiding in Him. **Righteousness will not fit well unless Jesus is your foundation.** Now you are ready to get dressed in righteousness to head outside. In a spiritual sense, this is the armor of God, the outer covering that protects you from the tactics of your enemy and accuser.

There are many spiritual outfits we can wear as believers: garments of praise, garments of salvation, wedding garments, robes of dedication, the covering of a cloak, and so on. Throughout Scripture, there are references to wearing, changing, putting on, or taking off different garments. These can represent many things, but they generally apply to an aspect of our character or actions and relate back to our relationship with God. Garments in Scripture may have a negative connotation, such as filthy garments. You can learn a lot from an in-depth study on this topic, but for now, our focus will be on those things that we are instructed to put on or put off in the New Testament.

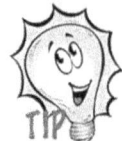

The Wardrobe

When you dress well, people take notice. The same is true when it comes to your spiritual "clothing." Your armor becomes a witness of Christ to the world. Your completed wardrobe prepares you to experience the abundant life God promises. Fully dressed, you live in peace, allow your faith to grow, cling to the Word, hold firm to your salvation, love the truth, and pursue righteousness. Now you are ready to be God's ambassador, representing Him in freedom.

Your Wardrobe with Christ

➤ Put off your old self (your flesh) and put on your new self (the likeness of Christ).

Do not lie to one another, seeing that you have put off the <u>old self with its practices</u> and have <u>put on the new self</u>, which is being renewed in knowledge <u>after the image of its creator</u>. (Colossians 3:9 – 10)

To <u>put off your old self</u>, which belongs to your former manner of life and is corrupt through deceitful desires, and to be renewed in the spirit of your minds, and to <u>put on the new self, created after the likeness of God</u> in true righteousness and holiness. (Ephesians 4:22 – 24)

➤ Dress yourself in Christ each day.

For as many of you as were baptized into Christ have <u>put on Christ</u>. (Galatians 3:27)

But <u>put on the Lord Jesus Christ</u>, and make <u>no</u> provision for the flesh, to gratify its desires. (Romans 13:14)

➤ Put off sin and the passions, temptations, and old practices of the flesh.

Therefore <u>put away all filthiness and rampant wickedness</u> <u>and receive</u> with meekness <u>the implanted word</u>, which is able to save your souls. (James 1:21)

So <u>put away all malice</u> and <u>all deceit</u> and <u>hypocrisy</u> and <u>envy</u> and <u>all slander</u>. (1 Peter 2:1)

Therefore, having <u>put away falsehood</u>, let each one of you speak the truth with his neighbor, for we are members one of another. (Ephesians 4:25)

The night is far gone; the day is at hand. So then let us <u>cast off the works of darkness and put on the armor of light</u>. (Romans 13:12)

➤ Put **on** love, light, the new self, godly character, and virtues.

Put on then, as God's chosen ones, holy and beloved, compassionate hearts, kindness, humility, meekness, and patience. (Colossians 3:12)

And above all these <u>put on love</u>, which binds everything together in perfect harmony. (Colossians 3:14)

For in this tent we groan, longing to <u>put on our heavenly dwelling</u>, if indeed by putting it on we may not be found naked. For while we are still in this tent, we groan, being burdened—not that we would be unclothed, but that we would <u>be further clothed</u>, so that what is mortal may be swallowed up by life. For in this tent we groan, longing to put on our heavenly dwelling. (2 Corinthians 5:2)

➤ Put on your full set of armor so you can stand firm and not give the enemy a place.

> *Therefore take up the whole armor of God, that you may be able to withstand in the evil day, and having done all, to stand firm. Stand therefore, having fastened on the belt of truth, and having put on the breastplate of righteousness, and, as shoes for your feet, having put on the readiness given by the gospel of peace. In all circumstances take up the shield of faith, with which you can extinguish all the flaming darts of the evil one; and take the helmet of salvation, and the sword of the Spirit, which is the word of God, praying at all times in the Spirit, with all prayer and supplication. (Ephesians 6:13 – 18)*

It is often difficult to do right; the battle with our flesh is real. Paul told us in 1 Corinthians 9:27, *"But I discipline my body and keep it under control, lest after preaching to others I myself should be disqualified."* The word Paul used for discipline implies he is beating his flesh black and blue to keep it under control so as not to damage his witness for Christ.

> *And let us not grow weary of doing good, for in due season we will reap, if we do not give up. (Galatians 6:9)*

Questions to Ponder

42.6) Do you have a constant back-and-forth struggle between living for Christ and living for your flesh? Describe your own struggle with your flesh.

42.7) What thoughts or feelings may cause you to give place to the enemy?

42.8) Is there something you hold as an idol above God? (This could be a person, desire, ideal, thought, emotion, or stronghold.)

42.9) Is there sin in your life that you keep returning to? What do you need to "put off"?

42.10) Considering your progress, what do you still need to "put on" to replace old hang-ups?

In your Journal, record potential future stumbling-blocks that you may have discovered in this lesson.

What spiritual clothing will you dress in to replace old beliefs and habits?

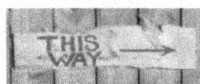

Your coach has an activity for you this week.

When Christ died for our sins, he took everything of our old self. It was not just sins nailed to that cross, but the result of our sin nature. Your shame, pride, anger, insecurity, anxiety, pain, depression, and labels no longer belong to you. They died on the cross with Jesus. His death made all things new. One day, we will fully transform into Christ's likeness, and there will be no trace of our sin nature left.

Look for sins, pride, control, negativity. Listen for times when you say or think, "I am _____." Each time you are rejecting who you are, remember the I AM placed your "bad" on His shoulders to be crucified with Him.

Chapter Seventeen

Choosing Healthy Relationships

A Very Important Chapter!

Why Focus on Relationships?

Relationship is the key to recovery. Relationship with God foremost, then relationship with self, and now relationships with others. Think back on your journey. You are likely to discover most of your trouble and pain originated **directly or indirectly** with other people. It is vital to build healthy relationships, identify toxic behaviors, communicate well, and handle conflict biblically **to prevent falling away from God and relapse.**

Healthy, caring relationships add a rich blessing to your life. Challenging times are not so difficult when you have someone by your side. Yet the most tender, loving relationships can cause you the most pain when you feel betrayed, rejected, or left behind by your loved one(s). Unavoidable pain is part of this life. Jesus understands these hurts, as He too experienced rejection, betrayal, and loss. **He helps you through these situations.** You are not alone.

Relationships can be toxic or dysfunctional. God's Word gives you all the aid you need to avoid or navigate these types of relationships. **The people with whom you associate matter to God and to your recovery.** People have a significant influence in your life and may lead you to question your value and worth. Toxic people dump their burdens on your shoulders, judge you, lie to you, reject you, harm you, and use and manipulate you. The effects of another's sin have a far reach, often right into your heart.

Through this journey, you have learned how important it is to love yourself. You understand that your worth and value are inherent to you, not dependent on your success or another's opinions of your worth. This alone is a powerful aid to building healthy relationships. One of Satan's greatest tools is your fear of rejection and shame. **Without that influence, the fear of man loses its power**, and God's voice becomes clear. Healthy boundaries help you identify and cut loose from the bondage of toxic relationships. Effective communication makes misunderstandings less likely to cause pain and division.

People's words and actions affect our lives. The way you deal with life issues either makes you victorious or destroys you. Handling conflict God's way will insulate you from the negative effects of people-problems while developing a Christ-like character in you and keeping you safe. **Engaging in healthy conflict is a way to show love to yourself.** The objective of recovery is **not to avoid pain and conflict.** Rather, the goal is to walk through your trials confident in God's protection.

You can have confidence in God's help. Recall Jesus' prayer for His believers in John 17:

> *I have given them your word, and the world has hated them because they are not of the world, just as I am not of the world. I do not ask that you take them out of the world, but that you keep them from the evil one. (John 17:14 – 15)*

Lesson 43 — Circles of Relationship

Nothing feels more rewarding than a healthy relationship, or more devastating than an unhealthy one. Are you pursuing a friendship with someone who should be an acquaintance? We long for close, real companionship, for another person to fully know us, but Jesus should fill those needs first. Moving forward with Christ may mean reevaluating your relationships.

Relationship is the giving of your heart to another. Therefore, this lesson defines relationship by how much you <u>trust another with your heart</u> and <u>not by marital or blood relation</u>.

What Is a Friend?

In our culture, we often call anyone we know a friend. Friends may be related to you, but not all your relatives are your friends. Scripture warns us about having too many people we call friends. You may have 500 or 1,000 friends on social media, but are they authentic friendships? Most people we call friend we should really consider acquaintances.

A man of many companions may come to ruin, but there is a friend who sticks closer than a brother. (Proverbs 18:24)

Throughout Scripture, examples of friendship share one commonality: They are all sacrificial relationships. True friends are rare. You may have only one person in your life that you could consider a genuine friend. A friend lays down his or her right to retribution, to be self-seeking, and hide behind walls. A friend knows your innermost you. They show loyalty, devotion, and dependability. A friend gives wise counsel that leads you to the Lord and righteousness. They will ***not*** always agree with you, and they do not smother you in flattery. These are the people you want in your inner circle.

This level of friendship bears lasting fruit. Examples in Scripture show that friendship is the greatest connection, the greatest love you can have for another person. Friendship is reciprocal and sacrificial. One beautiful illustration of friendship in Scripture is that of Jonathan and David. The Lord knit their souls together. What hurt one hurt the other. What rejoiced one gave joy to the other. They would sacrifice for one another, even to their own detriment.

As soon as he had finished speaking to Saul, the soul of Jonathan was knit to the soul of David, and Jonathan loved him as his own soul. (1Samuel 18:1)

Scripture shows us another such friendship in the relationship between Naomi and her daughter-in-law, Ruth. After the death of their husbands, Naomi directed Ruth to return to her people to protect her from a life of hardship. Ruth refused to go, showing loyalty to Naomi, and illustrating a friendship forged in the love of God.

*But Ruth said, "Do not urge me to leave you or to return from following you. For where you go I will go, and where you lodge I will lodge. Your people shall be my people, and your God my God. Where you die I will die, and there will I be buried. May the L*ORD *do so to me and more also if anything but death parts me from you. (Ruth 1:16 – 17)*

The reward of genuine friendship is two lives knitted together and love greater than any other relationship, apart from the love of Jesus. Friendship is not just about what one does for or gives to the other. **Friends reciprocate with selfless love, joy, trust, belonging, companionship, and loyalty, sharing their lives, and being known by one another.**

What Is an Acquaintance?

Most of your relationships may not fit this definition of friendship. Instead, they are probably acquaintances. These are folks you interact with on a regular basis but **cannot trust with the innermost parts of your heart.** An acquaintance may be a relative, or someone with whom you minister, work, or socialize, but **lack a reciprocal or sacrificial relationship.**

The Q Chart

The Q chart shows circles of relationship by how close a person is to your heart. Your most trusted and closest people are the smallest circles nearest to your heart. **The nearer a person is to your heart, the more vulnerable you become.** Yet these are the most rewarding relationships. Notice that **the closer it gets to your heart, the smaller the circle is.** Larger circles represent more people than the smaller circles.

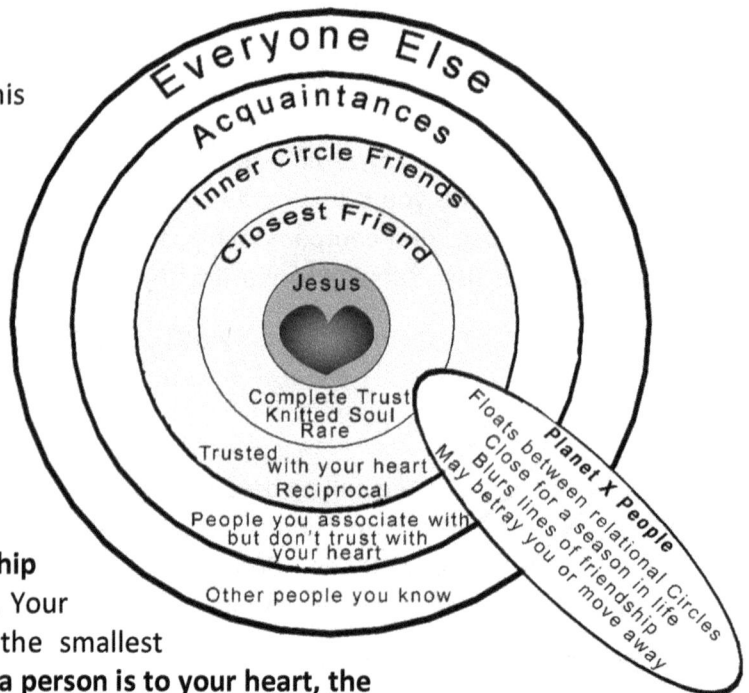

Here is what these circles represent:

- The shaded area represents your inner circle.

- The center circle represents your heart, and **the only one** who fits in the circle with your heart **is Jesus.** He has full access to your heart and is your first and closest friend.

- The closest friend circle has the **one** closest friend that you **absolutely trust** with your heart. This **may or may not** be a spouse or family member. This relationship represents mutual "best friendness." Having multiple people in this circle is difficult, and in most cases impossible, to maintain.

- Your next circle is your inner circle friendships. It contains certain friends or family members you **trust with your heart** but are not as close to as the person in the previous ring. They must be trustworthy, people you feel safe to confide in, and who share the same level of trust in you. **Relatives in this circle must also meet this criterion.**

- Then you have acquaintances. These are friends and relatives you spend time with for a variety of reasons. You may enjoy their company very much, but you do not give them **the same level of trust** as your inner circle friendships, **or the trust does not extend both ways.**

- The last circle contains **everyone else** you know, but with whom you lack any significant interactions.

- Then there are what we call the "Planet X People" because they break orbit. They float in and out of the different circles. **These relationships are short-term.** These folks impact your life for a season or for specific reasons. They may move away, grow distant, travel a different path in life, lack the loyalty to stick around. They may even use or betray you.

- Strangers are outside of the circle.

Not Everyone Should Be a Friend

Genuine friendship requires **vulnerability**, and that is frightening for many people. People who have been hurt, rejected, used, or manipulated fear openness with others. Yet we rob ourselves of one of the greatest gifts God gives when we live with our hearts guarded.

The Lord knows the risk of opening our hearts and lives to another person, which is why **He warns us to use wisdom when choosing our friends** and warns against allowing the influence of dishonest, manipulative, or negative people into our inner circles. Friendship is always mutual. No one should coerce you into a friendship. Likewise, if your investment in someone is not reciprocated, reconsider the relationship.

One who is righteous is a guide to his neighbor, but the way of the wicked leads them astray.
(Proverbs. 12:26)

Healthy Friendships

Look at what defines a healthy friendship. Are your relationships healthy?

- **Mutual Choice** – Friendship is not one-sided, chosen for you, or coerced through guilt or intimidation.
  "Two are better than one, because they have a good reward for their toil" (Ecclesiastes 4:9)

- **Mutual Benefit** – A friendship is reciprocal, not codependent. In a reciprocal relationship, both people benefit from mutual acts of love and companionship. Codependent relationships give a perceived benefit based on need or fear instead of from an overflow of genuine love.
  "Bear one another's burdens, and so fulfill the law of Christ" (Galatians 6:2).

- **Mutual Respect** – In a healthy friendship, each person respects the other's individuality. They accept on another's differences and decisions. They are not jealous, controlling, or judgmental, but are quick to overlook faults, give grace, and forgive generously.
  "Do nothing from selfish ambition or conceit, but in humility count others more significant than yourselves" (Philippians 2:3).
  "Love one another with brotherly affection. Outdo one another in showing honor" (Romans 12:10).

- **Mutual Concern** – Friends know each other intimately and will share their lives with one another. They hurt for one another's hurts and rejoice over one another's victories.
  "Let each of you look not only to his own interests, but also to the interests of others"
  (Philippians 2:4).

- **Mutual Beliefs** – Friends must share the same beliefs. You cannot walk through life with someone who is taking a different road.
  "Complete my joy by being of the same mind, having the same love, being in full accord and of one mind" (Philippians 2:2).
  "What accord has Christ with Belial? Or what portion does a believer share with an unbeliever?"
  (2 Corinthians 6:15).

- **Mutual Growth** – Friends grow together and make one another better. If you are the smartest person you know, it is time to acquire different friends.
  "Iron sharpens iron, and one man sharpens another" (Proverbs 27:17).
  "And let us consider how to stir up one another to love and good works" (Hebrews 10:24).

- **Mutual Trust** – Friends are open and truthful when they make mistakes, offend someone, or make poor choices. They put your wellbeing above their risk of rejection.
  "Faithful are the wounds of a friend, but the kisses of an enemy are deceitful" (Proverbs 27:6).

Examine the relationships in your life and the way you relate to others.

Answer the questions below, then fill out your own Q chart.

Questions to Ponder

Answer the questions below using this lesson's definitions of *friend* and *acquaintance*.

43.1) Describe the type of friend you are. How is the love of Christ evident in your friendships? Where is it missing in your friendships?

43.2) Are you the type of person you would want in your own inner circle? Why or why not?

43.3) How open are your friendships? Are your closest friendships superficial, or do you both see one another's inner man—the deepest part of who you are?

List everyone you interact with in person or on the internet. Include all relatives.
Use this list to answer the questions below and fill in the Q chart.

43.4) Examine your close friendships. What level of trust do you have for each person?

43.5) It is easy to see close relatives (spouse, children, parents, siblings) through a filter of your experiences with them, yet people change and grow. Examine these relationships. What level of trust do you give each person now?

43.6) Are family members in your inner circle only because they are family? Would they hold the same role in your life if they were not related? Why or why not?

43.7) Do you have people in your life who will keep you accountable and sharpen your faith (iron sharpening iron)?

43.8) What people in your life share your beliefs and theology?

43.9) Do you have a genuine friend?

43.10) What person (or people) in your life do you need to invest in more?

43.11) Whose influence in your life sways you away from the Lord or his commands?

43.12) Are there people to whom you should minister but keep out of your inner circle?

43.13) Which relationships should you reevaluate in your life?

43.14) Is there anyone in your life with whom you should not keep close company? Is there anyone you should avoid altogether?

43.15) Would those whom you consider in your inner circle say you are in their inner circle as well?

43.16) If those in your inner circle understood how this lesson defines friendship, would they say you fit that definition of a friend in their lives? Explain the ways you fit and do not fit that definition with each person.

43.17) Jesus is in your innermost circle. Would He say you reciprocate that level of friendship with Him?

Q Chart Worksheet

Fill in the Q chart. Add names of people in your life to the proper circle.
Who is in your inner circle? *(You may make copies of this page.)*

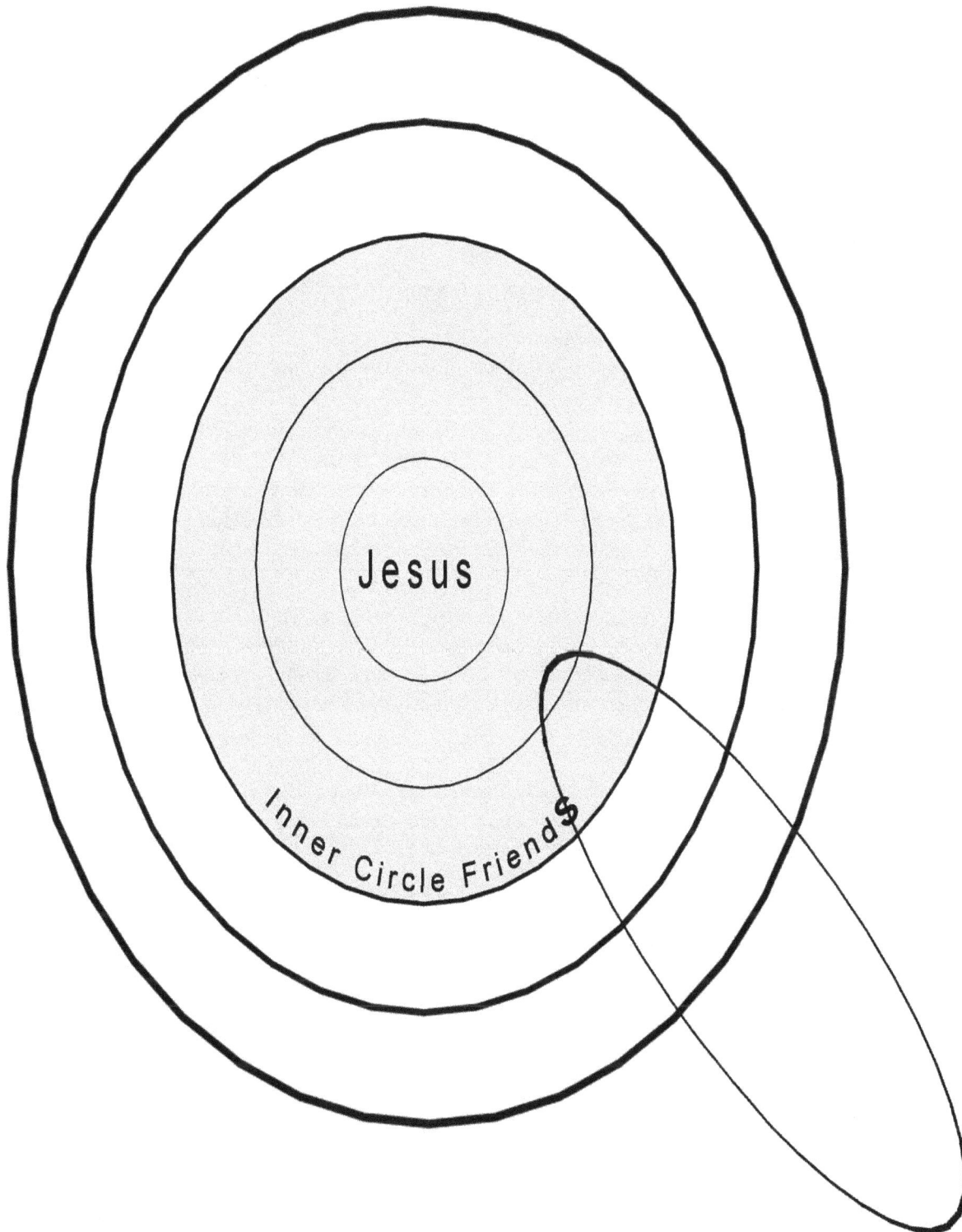

Jesus

Inner Circle Friends

Lesson 44 — Toxic Relationships & Behaviors

People may bless your life or be a detriment. Their opinions hold much less weight when you are confident in who you are. Even so, their toxic behaviors may harm you or lead you away from doing what is right with God. Scripture tells us to avoid such people.

As for a person who stirs up division, after warning him once and then twice, have nothing more to do with him, knowing that such a person is warped and sinful; he is self-condemned. (Titus 3:10 – 11)

Scripture defines many types of division. These can include harsh words and manipulation, causing dissention and quarrels, or arguments over theology. The Lord warns us to stay away from people who cause division and exhibit toxic behaviors. Their toxic behavior creates unhealthy and harmful relationships that pull us away from the journey God wants us to be on.

These are people the Lord warns us to stay away from:

- **Those who do evil or have wicked friends:** *"Blessed is the man who walks not in the counsel of the wicked, nor stands in the way of sinners, nor sits in the seat of scoffers"* (Psalm 1:1).

- **Those lacking self-control:** *"Make no friendship with a man given to anger, nor go with a wrathful man, lest you learn his ways and entangle yourself in a snare"* (Proverbs 22:24 – 25).
  Immoral people, especially those who claim to be Christians: "But now I am writing to you not to associate with anyone who bears the name of brother if he is guilty of sexual immorality or greed, or is an idolater, reviler, drunkard, or swindler—not even to eat with such a one"
  (1 Corinthians 5:11).

  "But understand this, that in the last days there will come times of difficulty. For people will be lovers of self, lovers of money, proud, arrogant, abusive, disobedient to their parents, ungrateful, unholy, heartless, unappeasable, slanderous, without self-control, brutal, not loving good, treacherous, reckless, swollen with conceit, lovers of pleasure rather than lovers of God, having the appearance of godliness, but denying its power. Avoid such people" (2 Timothy 3:1 – 5).

- **People with perverted speech:** *"Discretion will watch over you, understanding will guard you, delivering you from the way of evil, from men of perverted speech, who forsake the paths of uprightness to walk in the ways of darkness"* (Proverbs 2:11 – 13).

- **People who gossip and slander:** *"Whoever goes about slandering reveals secrets; therefore, do not associate with a simple babbler"* (Proverbs 20:19).

- **People prone to jealousy and selfish ambition**: *"For where jealousy and selfish ambition exist, there will be disorder and every vile practice"* (James 3:16).

- **Those who claim to be Christians but do not display the character of a Christian, or who have wrong teaching**: *"Do not be unequally yoked with unbelievers. For what partnership has righteousness with lawlessness? Or what fellowship has light with darkness?"* (2 Corinthians 6:14).

  "Beware of false prophets, who come to you in sheep's clothing but inwardly are ravenous wolves. You will recognize them by their fruits" (Matthew 7:15 – 16)

Associating with People to Witness

Jesus commands you to share the Gospel with all nations, not to make the world your friend. It can be tempting to bring someone into your circle of friends, thinking your positive influence will lead them to Christ. Unfortunately, Scripture warns us that this is not the case:

Do not be deceived: "Bad company ruins good morals." (1 Corinthians 15:33)

You therefore, beloved, knowing this beforehand, take care that you are not carried away with the error of lawless people and lose your own stability. (2 Peter 3:17)

Imagine, you are out for a walk and see a filthy dog. It is caked in mud, mangy, half its hair missing, and covered in flees. The dog is dying. With compassion, you bring the dog into your home and try to clean it up. You drench it in water, removing enough of the dirt that it encourages you to keep trying. You grab a clean white rag to remove the mud, and you attempt to remove the clumps of earth matted into the dog's fur and skin. The rag picks up dirt and moves it around but never truly gets the dog clean, and the rag becomes soiled. You wash the rag, but it is no longer white; now it is stained a grey-brown color. You apply a heavy-duty shampoo to the dog's fur, but it seeps into his sores, and he yelps and runs off. He loved the attention and tolerated the water, but he never desired to be clean. When the process hit a sore spot, anger and fear made the life-saving bath seem threatening.

In the above illustration the **dog is like a sinner** who needs Christ, filthy from sin, and in pain from deep wounds in his heart. The **water is like the Word of God** that you witness to the sinner. As it flows over the sinner, it gives hope and opens a door to God's healing. **The white rag represents your heart.** You let the sinner into your heart and life, hoping your godliness will be the influence that makes the difference. The sinner loves the attention, taking full advantage of it. You realize the filth embedded deep in him and tell the sinner he needs a relationship with the Lord—the shampoo. His flesh burns with fear and anger, and he leaves. You can only clean up the surface appearance. **Only the Lord can destroy the flesh and change a heart.** Meanwhile, the sinner's influence, words, and manipulation leave your heart stained.

The Takeaway

- We are supposed to share the Word, our testimony, and God's love with those in the world.

- Because of our sin nature, we must be diligent to protect what and who we allow to influence us.

- **We cannot make another righteous**, but they can influence us with evil.

- We represent God, but it is His job to draw people, save their soul, and change their heart.

- The Lord gives us discernment about who we should witness to and how.

Purity in Relationship

Who shall ascend the hill of the Lord? And who shall stand in his holy place? <u>He who has clean hands and a pure heart</u>, who does not lift up his soul to what is false and does not swear deceitfully. (Psalm 24:3 – 4)

One of the greatest temptations facing us is sexual temptation. It manifests in a variety of ways: lusting over another, watching sexual content in entertainment, sex outside of marriage, multiple or same-sex partners, or adultery. Because every sexual sin begins in our mind, this is our focus.

But I say to you that everyone who looks at a woman with lustful intent has already committed adultery with her in his heart. (Matthew 5:28)

Your sin begins the moment you look at salacious material or let your mind wander into titillating fantasies. It is the same as if you commit the acts you are fantasizing about. To protect your relationships, you must first guard your mind's purity.

To the pure, all things are pure, but to the defiled and unbelieving, nothing is pure; but both their minds and their consciences are defiled. (Titus 1:15)

For this is the will of God, your sanctification: that you abstain from sexual immorality; that each one of you know how to control his own body in holiness and honor, not in the passion of lust like the Gentiles who do not know God; that no one transgress and wrong his brother in this matter, because the Lord is an avenger in all these things, as we told you beforehand and solemnly warned you. <u>For God has not called us for impurity, but in holiness.</u> Therefore whoever disregards this, disregards not man but God, who gives his Holy Spirit to you.
(1 Thessalonians 4:3 – 8)

Protecting Purity

It is easy to fall into the trap of sexual sin, especially in your mind. Therefore, it is important to protect purity of mind and body, and the integrity of your marriage or future marriage.

How can a young man keep his way pure? By guarding it according to your word.
(Psalm 119:9)

The best guard against sexual sin is to **never give it room in your life**. Examine your motives and create reasonable boundaries. If you have a close friendship with someone of the opposite sex, consider how a new spouse may feel about that friendship. Protect your spouse; **do not tempt them to jealousy**.

Men and woman **do** need to interact in society, and this makes it important to create boundaries for your relationships. Examples of these boundaries may include not contacting anyone of the opposite gender privately or meeting with them alone behind closed doors. Create boundaries for your mind as well. Consider what people you meet with, where you go, and what you listen to or watch. Eliminate influences that cause your mind to wander where it should not.

Questions to Ponder

44.3) Have you ever let someone into your inner circle because you wanted to "fix" them or be a positive influence in their lives? What was the result?

44.4) What temptations or influences cause your mind to wander to impure thoughts?

44.5) What can you do to keep your thoughts pure?

44.6) Are there any boundaries you should create? How will you enforce them?

Lesson 45 — Hidden Dangers

> **IMPORTANT: Do not attempt to diagnose another person or yourself.**
>
> Often, people with destructive behavior experienced harm from their own trauma or dysfunctional relationships. However, do not attempt to diagnose another person or yourself. Instead, **use the terms in this lesson to identify the _toxic behaviors_** **in yourself or others that harm your relationships.**

The following lessons deal with some of the **most** toxic relationship dynamics. **It can be difficult to identify these dynamics in a relationship when you're in the midst of it, and it can be hard to leave the toxic environment.** The information below can help you spot hidden manipulation, control, and enabling, as well as false thinking passed down from past generations. If you believe you are in a damaging relationship, please let your coach know. They have additional resources and can guide you to **professional help**.

Codependency

Relationship is reciprocal by nature, meaning that both parties give to and receive from the relationship. Codependency distorts the reciprocal nature of a relationship. One person in the relationship meets his or her emotional needs (such as approval, worth, and value) by attempting to fix, enable, or mask another's unhealthy behavior. One is needy, the other needs to be needed. When Jesus fills all our needs, we are not dependent on another person to fill us. We become able to give to people out of an overflow of love. **Healthy relationships come from a desire to give oneself to another. Unhealthy relationships come from an attempt to fill a lack or a need.**

Codependent relationships prevent one or both parties from leading independent lives apart from the relationship. The relationship takes precedence over individual choices and pursuits. Codependency exists in most relationships where at least one of the people suffers from addiction, abuse, neglect, narcissism, or mental illness. The enabler sacrifices their individuality to care and cover for the dependent's physical or emotional issues.

Each person in a codependent relationship depends on the other's issues. Therefore, **healing one individual does not heal the relationship**. The strongholds no longer exist for the healed person, while the codependent continues to require that their needs to be met. **Both must heal or the relationship may not be sustainable.**

Codependency can exist between spouses, parents and children, friends, or coworkers. It is easy to live in denial about a codependent relationship, especially when you love the person or have made a significant investment in their life. Codependency may affect entire families, and toxic behaviors can be passed down to future generations. Codependent families often fear relying on outsiders, and they may hide or refuse to acknowledge problems in the family unit.

Gaslighting and Manipulation

Manipulation in a relationship destroys the one being manipulated. **Gaslighting is a particularly detrimental form of manipulation used to control and twist the reality of the victim.** The manipulator will lie or skew the facts of a situation to their benefit or to defeat the other person's argument. A gaslighter may reject any answer you offer to defend the truth and argue with you to a point of exhaustion.

People who are gaslighted question their reality: *Did I remember that wrong?* The perpetrator gains control through a consistent misrepresenting of facts to confuse the victim, making them believe they are stupid or crazy.

A person who gaslights often displays passive-aggressive behaviors. They may put unrealistic expectations on the other person or engage in an ongoing conflict if the person disagrees. They might neglect a person's needs until they get their desired result. Ghosting, shunning, or ignoring are also forms of passive-aggression.

This kind of manipulation in a relationship keeps you spinning. Your accuser may act angry at himself for hurting you in one moment, and the next minute he is blaming you. The confusion this causes creates a belief that you are not good enough. You may even begin to question, "What is wrong with me?" Not able to find the answers, you reject yourself and begin to lean on other people, including your abuser, to know how to be.

Healthy people communicate to be understood and to understand others. A gaslighter only seeks to prove that he is right and refuses to acknowledge a different perspective. Gaslighting feeds on a person's fear of the manipulator's rejection and desire for their approval.

The following lists do not diagnose any mental illness or disorder.

Signs of Codependency

*In the following lists, **note all frequent or recurring signs** in your relationships. If you feel unsafe, seek immediate help. Your coach has resources to help you.*

Do you, or does someone in your life:

- Spend all your energy meeting a person's needs and/or take responsibility for their happiness
- "Love" people that you can pity and rescue
- Feel trapped in a relationship
- Make most or all decisions
- Often rely on someone to decide for you
- Do most of the work to keep peace in a relationship
- Struggle to identify your feelings, or minimize, deny, or lie about how you feel
- Fear rejection or abandonment, or feel rejected if someone refuses your offer to help
- Engage in passive-aggressive behavior and/or consistent negativity
- Seek a sense of security and safety in someone else
- Hesitate to trust people
- Suffer low self-esteem or feelings of guilt or shame, or compare yourself with others

- Have difficulty saying "No"
- Struggle to sacrifice your own needs to please another
- Take responsibility for another person's wrong actions (i.e., apologizing for them, hiding their mistakes, or letting them off the hook)
- Defend and depend on the relationship, even at personal cost, believing it to be a selfless act
- Act over-sensitive or defensive in response to another's thoughts or feelings
- Violate boundaries, dictating the choices another person makes
- Have difficulty adjusting to change

Signs of Being Gaslighted

Do you:

- Have difficulty deciding because you do not trust yourself to make right choices
- Feel you lost yourself, or you remember yourself as a different person from who you are now
- Feel as if you cause another's misery
- Second-guess yourself, feel confused, or question your sanity
- Doubt things occurred the way you remember them or question your reality
- Often get accused of being too sensitive, wrong, insane, emotional, or overreacting
- Lie or make excuses because of fear of being criticized, attacked, or ridiculed
- Feel wrong and inadequate ("I should be a better spouse/friend/etc.")
- Apologize even when you feel you were wronged
- Fear something is wrong or threatening but cannot identify it
- Make excuses for another person's behavior

Questions to Ponder

45.1) **Thinking about past relationships and your childhood family, do you recognize any of the signs of codependency? State which relationship and give examples.**

45.2) **Thinking about current relationships, do you recognize any of the signs of codependency? State which relationship and give examples.**

45.3) **Do you recognize any sign that someone may be gaslighting you? Explain.**

45.4) **Give past and current examples of when you have been gaslighted.**

45.5) **Do you see yourself gaslighting others? Who do you gaslight and how? Give examples.**

*If you are in a manipulative or toxic relationship, **speak to your coach. He or she has additional resources available** for you and may direct you to professional help if needed.*

Lesson 46 — Dysfunction in the Family

The Dysfunctional Family Dynamic

When a family member has a mental illness, struggles with addiction, or is a narcissist, psychopath, or sociopath, it leads to a dysfunctional home environment. While these disorders may be different, the resulting dysfunction is similar. **Leave it to a professional to diagnose a mental disorder.** However, if you recognize the dynamics mentioned in this lesson in your current or childhood family, **seek the counsel of a mental health professional trained to deal with these disorders and the resulting trauma**.

Children growing up in a home with dysfunction may become adults who struggle with relationship issues. They often cannot figure out why they suffer from anxiety, depression, or other emotional symptoms. The following are lists of traits and roles commonly found in this dysfunctional family dynamic. **The level of dysfunction in the family depends on the degree of mental illness or abuse.** No family or relationship is the same as any other.

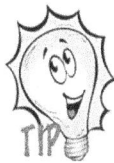

Many people who were in abusive relationships , especially in their childhood families end up in similar abusive relationships in adulthood. It is an environment they understand how to live in. They develop a subconscious belief that they deserve the abuse.

Often their **abuser defines love in a way that benefits the abuser and neglects the needs of the abused**. If this is you, it is vital to look at God's perspective of your value and love. It is difficult to break free from lies that you have spent your entire life believing. Submit these things to the Lord and have patience as He changes your heart to accept the truth.

Healthy vs. Unhealthy Family Roles

Members of a healthy family are interdependent. They assume roles within the **family community**, but these roles change as a child develops and different circumstances arise. This is a normal part of development, giving the child needed skills to live as an independent adult. There is no threat to the family dynamic when roles change, a family member dies, or a child leaves to start their own family.

In the **dysfunctional family, roles are co-dependent and more rigid.** Children bury part of their personality to stay in their role. This stifles emotional development and prevents learning healthy adult skills, such as coping with emotions and resolving conflicts. The dysfunctional family functions as **one entity, the family itself**, **not as individuals in a family community**. A person's role may change only if it meets the needs of the family. Someone leaving their role leaves a gap, which threatens the family's stability. Think of this family as one body, one individual. A person leaving or changing roles is like cutting out a major organ. It cripples the functioning ability of the family unit.

The Narcissistic Family

Narcissism is a rare diagnosis, but the impact of narcissistic abuse is not rare. Narcissism is a condition defined by a lack of empathy, an exaggerated belief in one's own self-importance, and the inability to admit wrongdoing. The narcissist proudly displays these beliefs in arrogant, patronizing, and demanding thoughts and actions. Narcissists manipulate others, thirst for approval and control, and are remarkably selfish. They **may play the victim** or seem untouchable.

Sometimes narcissistic behavior falls short of NPD (Narcissistic Personality Disorder). Any form or degree of narcissism or antisocial personality disorder creates an abusive environment that negatively impacts families. Bree Bonchay, LCSW, wrote a medically reviewed article in which he estimates narcissistic abuse affects half of the U.S. population in some way.[3]

Narcissistic abuse in the home creates a devastating family dynamic. Many adults suffer mental and emotional disorders resulting from the severe emotional abuse they endured as children, and **many find themselves in recovery programs**. The behaviors developed in a narcissistic family may transfer generationally, even if the children do not become narcissists. If you live in or come from a dysfunctional home, it is important to identify these toxic behaviors.

In this environment, children **must comply with the family narrative and value system or face rejection** from the family. The narcissist treats others as abnormal, like there is something wrong with them. This is manipulation. He creates insecurities and exploits people's strongholds to enforce control. The narcissist expects others to submit to his authority, even if it is wrong or abusive. He can read people's emotions and anticipate their responses, and he uses this information to guilt, shame, or coerce compliance. **Gaslighting is a favorite tool of the narcissist.**

Feelings of safety and security are absent in the home when a family member has narcissistic tendencies. Mistakes and accidents bring condemnation, whether or not a family member deserves guilt or admits his wrong. The family must hide abuse, often believing they are at fault for the abuse. Neglect and mistreatment create an atmosphere of continual fear in the home, but in public, the family puts on a good show, denying the truth of the life they are living, fearing the narcissist's ridicule, shame, and rage.

People living in a home with a true narcissist have difficulty escaping the environment without intervention. They usually do not have strong personalities, as the narcissist will work to prevent anyone close to them from having more power and influence than they do. When someone does stand up to a narcissist by establishing boundaries, the narcissist pushes or manipulates the boundaries, exhausting anyone trying to live free from their control.

Narcissistic families often exhibit pseudomutuality, which means that although the family is broken, they **appear** unified and tight-knit to the outside world. Disagreements become divisive and force family members to choose sides. Shame and ridicule are the cost of choosing the wrong side. Children may feel forced to choose between parents, siblings, or other family members who do not side with the narcissist. Only the narcissist may express their feelings, especially rage, discounting dissenting opinions and feelings and training others to suppress their emotional responses. In this kind of family, respecting one person requires that you disrespect another to keep up appearances. Love and respect are not available to everyone at once; some earn praise while others are shamed. The family roles in a narcissistic family change with the situation to maintain the family dynamic but not to benefit the individual.

---

[3] "Narcissistic Abuse Affects Over 158 Million People in the U.S.," *PsychCentral*, https://psychcentral.com/lib/narcissistic-abuse-affects-over-158-million-people-in-the-u-s/.

Traits of the Dysfunctional Family

- Children lack emotional access to parents. They do not feel heard, seen, or nurtured. Parents are judgmental and critical of their children.

- A narcissist may pit children against each other and compare them to one another. The parent may favor one child while another takes the brunt of his anger and frustration until the roles change. Siblings may grow up protecting one another, but more often they feel an emotional disconnect from one another.

- Children lack boundaries, or the boundaries change as the whim of the parent changes.

- Children learn negative messages about themselves through their parents' words and actions. They believe they are not good enough or are somehow defective. They believe they must earn their value by what they do instead of being valued for who they are.

- Children lack guidance, love, and direction from their parents. Instead, they serve the parents' emotional or physical needs, creating a distorted view of what love is.

- The family lacks respect for physical and emotional boundaries. No one has a right to privacy. Children learn unclear personal boundaries and never understand, even into adulthood, that family does not have the right to violate their privacy.

- Family members who cannot discuss their feelings experience multiple emotional issues. They believe the others consider their feelings unimportant, and they are too sensitive. The narcissist projects their own feelings onto others, and everyone else must repress their emotions, processing them in damaging ways.

- Family members experience emotional, psychological, and often physical abuse.

- The family keeps secrets. They must hide profound pain from the outside world and pretend nothing is wrong. The secrets become their reality.

- The family must maintain an image of perfection. Everything must seem better than it is. They worry about what friends, family, and neighbors will think of them.

- Effective communication skills are nonexistent in any sort of conflict. Unless presented as rage, there is no direct communication of an issue. It is easier to talk about another than to confront them, so the family often communicates through triangulation. This is when one person tells information about another to a third person, knowing, eventually, the person being talked about will hear it.

- Passive-aggressive behaviors create tension and an inability to trust other family members with your heart.

Roles in the Dysfunctional Family

Families suffering from addiction, mental illness, narcissism, and other forms of dysfunction have distinct family roles. Note that **seeing yourself in one of these roles does not necessarily indicate the type of dysfunction in your family**. Not all roles are present in all families.

A narcissistic parent's expectations may **force a child into a specific role**, or a child may **take on a specific role as a coping skill** or may **assume multiple roles**. Children suffering emotional abuse, like all children, need the attention and validation that are lacking in a dysfunctional environment. The family role that a child plays may continue into adulthood if he does not learn and apply healthy coping skills.

Key roles in the dysfunctional family

Read the two lists that follow, describing toxic behaviors and family roles. Note each role or sign that you recognize in your current or past relationships. Then answer the questions at the end.

- **The Focal Point** – The person, often a parent, to whom the family devotes their attention and energy. This role usually exists in a family where one or both parents have addiction, narcissism, psychopathy, or another personality disorder.

- **Orbiting Parent** – In a home where the focal point is one parent, the orbiting parent is the spouse. The children may be sympathetic as they see her as being treated unfairly by the other parent. Even so, the orbiting parent is too busy "orbiting" or appeasing the focal point to fully meet the children's needs.

- **The Golden Child** – The golden child can do no wrong. The focal point displays this child as a reflection of himself. He sees something about this child which gives him "bragging rights." The golden child believes that his value comes from what he does, and he perceives people less accomplished as having little value.

- **The Scapegoat Child** – The scapegoat is the child who does nothing right. He is the "bad seed" or "black sheep" of the family. He receives the brunt of a parent's anger, unrelenting blame, and **suffers humiliation in front of other family members**. The scapegoat is authentic and truthful about the family's issues and unjust behaviors. They may mean well but often act out in anger or rebellion in response to the injustice. The other family members expect the scapegoat to care about the family's needs, while treating them as if they have no needs of their own. Scapegoats do not receive the credit they deserve for their achievements, and they can never live up to their parents' expectations. They often have a deep-seated belief that they are incapable, worthless, and unloved.

- **Invisible/Lost Child** – This child is ignored because the parents are focused on their own issues and other children. The lost child **does not receive praise or blame** but is forgotten or treated as if they are invisible. Parents may care for the child's basic needs, but there is no investment in their life. These children learn basic life skills by watching siblings, and they become very independent. Believing they have no voice, they withdraw into their own little world. Lost children often struggle to feel like they fit in. They feel lonely, invisible, unloved, and unvalued.

Secondary Roles in dysfunctional families (Secondary roles may pair with key roles.)

- **The Dependent** – Dependents fall into a deep pit of substance abuse or dysfunction and face the most obvious challenges to recovery. The problem child, acting out in rebellion, is often a dependent. Everyone, including the dependent, realizes his behaviors must change. The family alters their behaviors to accommodate the dependent's lifestyle by enabling them and lying for them, willingly or unwillingly. Some may react by cutting off all contact with the dependent, which can change the entire family dynamic. The dependent must identify their unhealthy behavior and thought patterns to recover.

- **The Mastermind** – The mastermind is a manipulator and opportunist, often using coercion to get what he wants. This may is often a narcissist or he may be a dependent, using manipulation to continue or hide his substance use. Masterminds are self-absorbed, abusive, and driven by entitlement. A mastermind will intentionally confuse the family members to hide the truth about himself and his abuse. He will use and manipulate the rest of the family's dysfunction to his own benefit. He observes each person's behaviors and engages their dysfunctional role at will to achieve his intended purpose. He may create intentional conflict among family members to serve his interests. He knows how to use his charm to manipulate both the children and adults in the family. Masterminds may rebel or act like the scapegoat, engaging in their own form of misbehavior. They may take advantage of the caretaker's nature or use another enabler to get what they want. A mastermind is difficult to understand. His actions are despicable, but he creates chaos and takes advantage of people and opportunities, often to meet his own neglected needs.

- **Flying Monkey** – Like the flying monkeys in The Wizard of Oz, this enabler reports on and torments non-compliant family members—anyone who contradicts the "focal point," or anyone considered a threat to the family. Their unwavering loyalty to the family makes them easy to manipulate. The focal point uses the flying monkey's own issues to manipulate her to perpetrate abuse on his targeted victims through gaslighting, threats, guilt, shame, rejection, or violence. This clears the focal point of all wrongdoing. While the focal point is manipulating the flying monkey to do his dirty work, he may also be manipulating the target by acting selfless or as a temporary martyr to gain deeper trust and commitment from them.

- **The Mascot** – The mascot is the family joker, using humor and antics to relieve the stress in the home. Their jokes are often insensitive or immature. They tend to be the center of attention and popular because of their "class clown" antics. Mascots cannot deal with the feelings of powerlessness that arise from conflict, violence, anger, or other negative family situations. They use humor to communicate repressed emotions; to hide deep insecurity; to avoid conflict rather than address issues; and to escape difficult emotions like pain, grief, anger, or fear. Humor becomes the mascot's identity. She has many superficial friends but is unable to sustain a deep relationship. She cannot let anyone see the person behind her jester mask. The mascot stays too busy to stop and think, attempting to avoid the depression and anxiety that come in the quiet. She may have difficulty concentrating, leading to problems in school or at a job. The mascot is a people-pleaser, so her adult relationships are often codependent.

191

- **Caretaker** – This family member is an enabler who covers up or makes excuses for the issues of the addict/narcissist. She becomes the family martyr, taking care of the addict/narcissist's responsibilities, and protecting him from the consequences of his actions or taking them upon herself. The caretaker seeks to be the emotional rescuer for the rest of the family but neglects her own emotional support. She expresses sensitivity to emotion and often seems calm and caring. A caretaker bases her self-worth and identity on her ability to help the family. She shows her concern with nurturing support, listening, consoling, protecting, and advising family members, yet her efforts to save the family enforce each person's codependent roles. Caretakers are people-pleasers and problem-fixers—that is, they solve everyone's problems but their own. They have everyone's answers, but do not know how to care for themselves. They give love, but do not know how to receive it, and they may push genuine love away. Caretakers often experience trauma bonding with the narcissist. In adulthood, they often have **highly toxic codependent relationships, which become one-sided and abusive**. They tend to become everyone's doormat.

- **Hero** – The hero wants to present a "normal" family appearance. This is the perfectionist who, like the caretaker, covers up family secrets. The hero takes responsibility for the family image and becomes the true mask of a dysfunctional family. Heroes suppress their own emotions so much that they are unable to experience most emotions at all. Their insecurity drives them to be accomplished and successful, seeking achievement in any form possible. The hero is often the older sibling, but not always. The hero is stuck in his ways, the self-appointed responsible one, who expects perfection—from himself and others—to maintain the family image. He appears to be the most successful, "together" person in the family, but accomplishments do not satisfy his needs. Heroes suffer from their high expectations and stress levels and develop major control issues to avoid feeling guilt and shame from failure. They place blame on other family members for their family's issues creating volatile relationships in the home, but sometimes people outside of the home bear the brunt of the blame. Their family's problems become the fault of whoever benefits the hero's narrative.

> ### Questions to Ponder
>
> 46.1) Do the people in your family (whether now or in the past) have roles that are interdependent or codependent? Do the roles respect individuality? Explain your answers.
>
> 46.2) Do you recognize any of the traits of a dysfunctional family from your childhood family or other past relationships? Explain and give examples.
>
> 46.3) Do you recognize any of the traits of a dysfunctional family in your current relationships? Explain and give examples.
>
> 46.4) Thinking about your childhood family and past relationships, can you see yourself or other family members in dysfunctional family "roles"? Explain and give examples.
>
> 46.5) Thinking about your current family dynamic, do you see yourself or other family members that fit in a specific role? Explain and give examples.
>
> *If you are stuck in a manipulative or toxic relationship, <u>speak to your coach for more help.</u>*

Lesson 47 — Insist on Healthy Relationships

Movies and television shows often depict people with personality disorders as mass murderers capable of an insane amount of harm. This makes entertaining fiction, but actual people rarely act this way. In real life, people suffering from personality disorders may not show the outward signs you might expect. For example, a covert narcissist may act passive, give fake apologies, be quiet, or seem like the victim. A psychopath **may** be violent but **will** cause emotional and psychological harm. Having multiple disorders may compound a person's dysfunction.

It is important to recognize damaging behaviors, but do not make your own diagnoses. Someone who exhibits any of these behaviors needs professional, godly help from a therapist **trained to deal with these disorders**. A person without training **cannot diagnose them or fix them**. Remember, most people's dysfunctional behaviors arise from significant pain and insecurity. Please do not try to change them. Instead, examine their behavior and **change your own** to protect yourself from harmful situations.

Protecting Yourself from Dangerous Relationships

Instead of focusing on the poor behavior of another, focus on yourself. You cannot control what people do, but you can control how you respond to their words and actions. **Confidence in your own identity, loving yourself, and knowing healthy relationship dynamics** can prevent a negative or dysfunctional person from abusing you.

Shame

A person riddled with shame is a prime target for manipulation and abuse. This is why it is vital to know your value and identity as a child of God. You cannot have confidence to step out of dysfunction if a little voice inside you whispers that you deserve the abuse. You cannot fight the lies of dysfunction without a healthy love for yourself. Remind yourself of the truth found in God's Word: The guilts and shame of the past no longer belong to you. Love the person you are in Christ, love the new creation you are becoming, and have confidence that God will finish the work He started in you. Know without doubt that you are worth treating well because your creator says you are. **Love yourself enough to stand up for yourself. The way people treat you matters as much as how you treat them.** Their words do not define you. Stand firm in the truth.

> *Fear not, for you will not be ashamed; be not confounded, for you will not be disgraced; for you will forget the shame of your youth, and the reproach of your widowhood you will remember no more. (Isaiah 54:4)*

> *Bless the Lord, O my soul, and forget not all his benefits, who forgives all your iniquity, who heals all your diseases, who redeems your life from the pit, who crowns you with steadfast love and mercy. (Psalm 103:2 – 4)*

Shame, especially when it has been embedded in your heart since childhood, is difficult to overcome. Like everything else in recovery, it is a process. Speak with your coach about areas of shame you still hold on to. Look for any problematic thinking patterns that remain and remind yourself daily of who you are and who you are becoming. The more you bring lies into the light, the less power they have.

Understand Healthy Relationships

Understanding healthy relationships helps you identify how people should fit into your life. Regardless of the relationship, every person should treat you with respect.

Healthy Relationship	Unhealthy Relationship
➢ Each person values the relationship equally.	➢ The relationship feels one-sided.
➢ Each person respects the other as an individual outside the relationship.	➢ At least one person feels they may not have a life outside the relationship.
➢ Neither person feels other friendships threaten the relationship.	➢ Jealousy causes control or manipulation of the other person's friendships.
➢ Each person supports the other's hobbies, interests, and other pursuits.	➢ One tries to control the decisions of the other or makes all the decisions for them.
➢ Each person shares their lives, interests, and pain. If you know another fully, you know and care about what hurts them.	➢ They share common interests and activities but have no desire or ability to share the deep matters of their heart or their pain.
➢ Both people are honest and truthful.	➢ Lies and manipulation are common.
➢ Each person is free to express an opposing viewpoint.	➢ One or both people ridicule and dismiss opposing viewpoints.
➢ Both people trust one another with their flaws and innermost secrets.	➢ Both people put up walls to guard their hearts.
➢ Each person bears the other's burdens and considers the best interests of the other.	➢ One person dismisses the other's needs, expecting his own needs to take precedence.
➢ Each person has access to material and financial assets.	➢ Money is a means to control and manipulate.
➢ Each person overflows love into the other.	➢ The relationship is built on need, not love.
➢ Both people treat each other with kindness and understanding.	➢ One or both people treat the other with contempt and ridicule.
➢ Each person is gracious, overlooking the other's faults and mistakes and helping them overcome.	➢ One or both people believe that a person can never be better than their mistakes and faults.
➢ Communication is open and honest and allows a healthy expression of feelings.	➢ Those in the relationship cannot communicate their feelings without worrying about insults and ridicule.
➢ Both people feel heard when sharing their thoughts and feelings.	➢ At least one person feels like the other never hears them, or like their words do not matter.
➢ Both people can offer and receive correction in a disagreement, stick to the subject, have self-control, admit wrongdoing, and problem-solve to find resolution.	➢ In a disagreement, one person faces ridicule and condemnation as the other attempts to cover up wrongdoing and shut down the conversation. The goal is not resolution.
➢ Both are walking together with the Lord.	➢ The people in the relationship are on different spiritual paths.
➢ In a marital relationship, each person feels safe and comfortable with the sexual activity.	➢ One person in the marriage pressures or forces the other to engage in sexual activity they are not comfortable with.

If your relationship(s) has a few unhealthy characteristics, you can work to correct damaging behaviors. However, when a person is **unwilling to communicate, recognize, or change their behavior**, it may be time to end the relationship. When you cannot distance yourself from a relationship, you must set boundaries.

Boundaries

Boundaries are not a means of control or manipulation. Boundary-setting is not a passive-aggressive behavior that withholds communication, finances, or love until the other person complies with your will. You are not forcing someone to agree with you or do things your way. Boundaries protect you from abuse. Creating distance or boundaries gives you the space you need to heal.

Creating healthy boundaries in a relationship involves **defining clear rules** about what you will not allow in your life and **consistent enforcement** of those rules. You should implement some boundaries with everyone you interact with. Make the rules fit your circumstances. Bear in mind that it is in our flesh to push boundaries and bend rules. **Bendable rules mean breached boundaries.**

Manipulators attempt to find ways around boundaries. They might try to convince you that you are wrong for creating boundaries in the first place, or trick you into dropping boundaries altogether. You may need separation to establish healthy boundaries. If you cannot cut off contact, create distance and limit interaction. Prepare to walk out of the room or stop communication the moment a person violates one of your rules.

Essential Rules for Every Relationship

"You will respect me." Tolerate no ridicule, name-calling, insults, gaslighting, manipulation, guilt trips, or false accusations. End the conversation immediately.

"You will respect my time. I am not obligated to your time frame." Do not feel guilty about making someone wait for your schedule to be free. You can respect their desires so long as you realize that your life does not revolve around their schedule.

"You will respect my words. When I say no, the answer is no." Do not allow others to pressure you to do something that violates your boundaries or morals, or that makes you uncomfortable. It is okay to refuse to help someone. You know the amount of responsibility you can handle. It is your right to consider your own needs.

"You will respect my privacy." Do not allow another to violate your online or offline privacy. Your home, belongings, conversations, body, and life are your business. Spying on you, following you, asking others about you, going through your phone or journals, or talking/gossiping about you are never acceptable behavior.

"You will respect my choices." It is not your responsibility to meet another's expectations, (except perhaps when performing your job, or when you choose to commit to a responsibility). Set reasonable expectations for yourself and live by those standards. You are free to make your own choices in life.

"If you have a problem with me, come to me directly." Triangulation is not acceptable. If someone takes issue with you, they should address it with you and not gossip to another about the issue.

Questions to Ponder

47.1) Do you feel shame from any of the relationships in your life? Which words or actions make you feel shameful, and who causes those feelings?

47.2) Looking at the traits of healthy and unhealthy relationships, how do you feel about the quality of your close relationships?

47.3) Examine the relationships with the greatest impact on your life. Are there unhealthy behaviors in these relationships? List them.

47.4) You should have healthy boundaries in every relationship. Which relationships consistently violate healthy boundaries?

47.5) Do you feel trapped in a relationship with mental or physical abuse? Do you feel unheard, ridiculed, or gaslighted? Describe these relationships.

47.6) Abusive relationships require stronger boundaries. Review the information *on the next pages* about establishing and enforcing healthy boundaries. Then make a plan.

If you believe you are in a toxic mentally or physically abusive relationship, ask your coach to direct you to professional help.

Obviously, **it is easier to avoid a toxic or abusive relationship** than to deal with one you are already in. How you handle this depends on your situation. If a person's abuse is a stumbling block to you following the Lord or His will for your life, choose the Lord first. **The next few pages give guidelines to establish healthy boundaries in relationships.**
Do not think that I have come to bring peace to the earth. I have not come to bring peace, but a sword. For I have come to set a man against his father, and a daughter against her mother, and a daughter-in-law against her mother-in-law. And a person's enemies will be those of his own household. Whoever loves father or mother more than me is <u>not worthy of me</u>, and whoever loves son or daughter more than me is <u>not worthy of me</u>. And whoever does not take his cross and follow me is <u>not worthy of me</u>. Whoever finds his life will lose it, and <u>whoever loses his life for my sake will find it</u>. (Matthew 10:34 – 39)

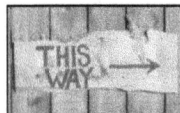

> Your coach has additional resources to help you learn, establish, and enforce healthy boundaries.

Enforcing Boundaries

In a dysfunctional or narcissistic family dynamic, **your boundaries are seen as a threat and will be met with resistance**. Those threatened by your boundaries may attempt to manipulate you, **dictate your choices**, or **isolate** you from people who speak a narrative different from theirs. **They may ridicule you, lay guilt on you, say they cannot live without you, or warn that they will do something drastic if you leave.** They may **intimidate**, **threaten**, or make it seem like **you are in the wrong**. If an abuser ignores or encroaches upon your boundaries, you must enforce your boundary with consequences. However, sometimes a broken person with a repentant heart is working with God to change toxic behaviors. As their behavior changes, you may modify the original boundaries.

Here are the key things to remember when setting boundaries:

❖ **God defines you; the abuser does not.** Do not allow anyone to tell you who you are or define your character or your intelligence. An abuser may accuse you of something they are doing. For example, if they are gossiping, they may accuse you of spreading gossip. Do not allow anyone to define your actions or motives.

❖ **You are not on trial. Do not give a defense.** An abuser may scrutinize your actions and lob false accusations at you. Do not allow intimidation to cause you to second guess what you know is true or right. **In a relationship in which you do not trust your heart to an abuser, you do not owe him an explanation or need to justify your thoughts, feelings, or actions.** The abuser gains a sense of power and control when he pushes your buttons. He feels superior when dissecting your perceived poor qualities. He may judge every word you say while accusing you of being judgmental. **You cannot win in this scenario.** Refuse to take part. Keep your mind focused on truth and stop accusations and insults immediately by walking away.

❖ **You have the power!** You have control and power over your choices, your feelings, and your thoughts. You are allowed to feel your feelings, think your own thoughts, and make your own choices. Even if your choices are bad, they are your mistakes to make. A controlling person tries to disempower you by making you feel bad for your choices or insisting you do things their way. Remember, you are an individual with your own mind. Other people will not experience the consequences of your actions; **you will**. Make your choices based on what you believe is best for your own life with the Lord's leading.

❖ **Avoid sharing personal information.** An abuser loses any right to details about your life or feelings. **They will use this information against you.** Keep conversations to mundane topics like the weather or news. If you must share a decision, avoid discussing the reason behind your choice. An abuser may draw you in with a need. Be unavailable. You do not need to explain yourself. Stay uninvolved. When drama or gossip is the topic being discussed, do not share your advice, opinions, or problem-solve. An abusive person may use your goodwill to violate your boundaries or to drag you into another's personal drama.

❖ **Plan to avoid manipulation.** Keep separate finances. Stop gaslighting and turn it back on them with the truth. Do not allow them to drive you to anger. Walk away from the "silent treatment." Plan a response to a manipulator's **FOG tactic** (fear, obligation, and guilt), which he may use against you. **Plan and practice** ways to enforce your boundaries and responses to the person's manipulation tactics.

Use the following suggestions to prepare yourself to enforce boundaries:

❖ **Prevent manipulation.** When you set boundaries, your abuser will pull out all the stops. Manipulation can seem like your own thoughts, making it exceedingly difficult to identify. The abuser may minimize your feelings while blaming you for how much you have hurt them. They act innocent, as if **they are the victim** of your anger, or accuse you of being sensitive or emotional.

To help identify manipulation, use the acrostic **FOG: Fear, Obligation, and Guilt**. This is a tactic an abuser uses **to fog your mind and make it difficult for you to see the truth**. For example, an abuser may cause you to worry about him or the future (fear). He may make you feel obligated to speak to him or treat him differently (obligation). He may try to make you feel wrong for standing up for yourself or attack your perceived character flaws (guilt). This tactic is effective against people struggling with insecurity and shame. **Have confidence** in the Lord as a just protector, **believe in your identity in Christ**, and **stick with your plan** to escape the harm your abuser causes.

These are the key points to remember to prevent manipulation:

- Identify the manipulation the abuser uses.

- Remind yourself that your boundaries are not up for discussion.

- Remember to keep your emotions out of any conversation. Be diligent to observe your abuser's behavior and do not take it on yourself.

- Do not engage a question designed to lure you into a trap. Keep conversations brief.

- Do not talk about your personal choices or engage in conversations about their choices.

- If the abuser gives you the silent treatment, stop trying to communicate with them.

- Journal everything. Know what they said and how it made you feel. Keep records so you know the truth and are not manipulated by gaslighting attempts.

❖ **Remain steadfast.** An abuser attempts to test boundaries like a child seeing how far he can push a parent before getting a spanking. When you set boundaries, expect retaliation. You are in a battle for yourself. **If your borders are not solid, the abuser will breach them.** You are important, and you have a God-given purpose. Persevere. Do not give up on yourself or give in to the abuse.

❖ **Prepare your finances.** In a healthy marriage, you should take part in financial decisions and partake in the family income with your spouse. Separate your finances, however, if your spouse seeks to control your spending, spend all the money, or keep money from you. Let him have his own money and take responsibility for yours. Separating your finances prevents an abuser from manipulating you with money.

❖ **Keep focused on yourself, not your abuser.** Keep your thoughts focused on your God, your rules, and your power over yourself. Don't waste precious time trying to get your abuser to understand how he hurt you; your explanations will likely fall on deaf ears. You may want him to care about you, or maybe you seek validation, but only the Lord can show him the truth. If he twists everything you say or do to validate himself, he will never hear or see you correctly. Constant rejection can make anyone question their value. Stop allowing an abuser to rob you of your value with their indifference and waste your time with fruitless effort. **You cannot change them, but you can alter your response!**

❖ **Prepare your emotions.** Does your abuser bring out the worst in you? We often become like the people we are around, especially picking up their negative traits. Remember our story about the dog? **When you reflect the abuser's behaviors**, such as criticizing, angry outbursts, or contempt, **he will ridicule you for your behavior**. This removes attention from him and places it on your "bad character." Building an emotional resistance to his actions will stop this cycle. You must have confidence. God says who you are, not your abuser.

Here are some key ways to master your emotions as you enforce your boundaries:

- **Do not internalize negative traits an** abuser projects on you. Recognize them as lies. For example, you may display anger, but that does not mean you are an angry person.

- **Understand your abuser.** Learn why they are behaving this way. What is their behavior, or your response to it, providing them? Realize the problem is with them and not you.

- **Watch, listen, and do not react.** You must stay calm and keep your emotions detached from the situation. Make a conscious decision to view your abuser as if from a distance. Observe what he does, as well as your behavior and responses. What can you learn about yourself and your abuser? Can you see manipulation tactics? What does it tell you about his character or yours? (Ask your coach for additional resources).

- **Do not reciprocate.** If an abuser responds in anger, do not show anger. Remove yourself from the situation. If he insults you, do not absorb or return the insult. When he is nice, say thank you, but do not give more. **No reaction means he has nothing to manipulate**.

- **Direct the conversation** back to the truth.

- **Remember your gratitude** for the blessings the Lord has provided and the work he has done in your life and keep your joy.

- **Advocate for yourself** the way you would for any other abused person.

❖ **Boundaries need consequences.** If an abuser violates your boundaries, prepare a consequence. It is vital that you be consistent, or your boundaries are worthless. A consequence may be to end a phone conversation, discontinue communication, leave a situation, or call the police. It is **your right and obligation to yourself to exit a destructive interaction**. You do not need approval or permission to leave or end communication. Your wellbeing is at stake. If your actions to enforce your boundaries jeopardize your physical safety, you may need to find shelter or involve the authorities.

❖ **Use preplanned, practiced responses.** Note how your abuser gets to you, and plan how you will respond to the situation. If a pat answer does not end the manipulation, stop the conversation immediately. State simple responses in a matter-of-fact tone.

- "The Lord uses my failure for my good."

- "I am confident in my choice."

- "No, you are interrupting me."

- "No, you may not speak to me that way."

- "No, that is not true."

- "Stop, you are disrespecting me." (Or manipulating me, discounting my feelings, etc.)

- "This is not constructive; I am ending this conversation." (Give no further explanation.)

Chapter Eighteen

Conflict Resolution

Lesson 48 — Conflict

The last chapter dealt with atypical situations found in serious dysfunction. **Conflict is not a dangerous concept in most situations.** In this chapter, we will learn about healthy conflict. First, let us review what we already learned.

- **Conflict** brings resolution and restoration. A **fight or quarrel** is a power struggle to prove your point, not a genuine attempt at reconciliation.

- **Search your heart** before engaging another in conflict. Is your anger justified? What is the other person's perspective? What could skew your perspective?

- **Go directly to the person** who sins against you and privately address the wrong. Do not seek validation of your emotions from a third party.

- **Be quick to address a matter** to give the devil no place to meddle in the situation. If someone has a problem with you, address the issue right away. As much as it depends on you, live at peace with everyone.

Why Engage in Conflict?

The easiest way through any issue is straight ahead. Always address a problem right away. It may make you sick just thinking about conflict, but **buried problems fester; they do not go away**. They escalate in your mind, so any reminder of the transgression brings back every hurt feeling.

Refusing to deal with an offense is unfair to you and to the one who offended you. They may be unaware of their offense or be responding to a hurt you caused them. Regardless of how much you love the other person, running away or refusing to communicate leaves unresolved pain for everyone involved, causing bitterness.

Agree to Disagree?

Have you ever heard someone say, "Let's just agree to disagree on this"? People think differently. Sometimes it is not worth breaking unity with another person to prove your point. This can be a good way to end frivolous arguments while respecting another's differences.

On the other hand, people often misuse "agreeing to disagree" to prevent someone with an opposing viewpoint from speaking their thoughts, to end uncomfortable conversations, to shift blame, or to avoid conflict altogether. This prevents ideas from being heard and **stops a conflict that may bring healing**. It is never okay to agree to disagree to avoid dealing with your wrongs or to allow another to avoid dealing with their wrongs toward you.

> ### Questions to Ponder
> **48.1) Do you notice a difference in the way you handle conflict now compared to the way you handled conflict before beginning your journey? Explain**

Questions to Ponder

48.2) What problems do you still have with conflict?

48.3) How do you avoid conflict or agree to disagree to keep peace in a situation?

To Judge or Not to Judge

When conflict arises, people may accuse you of judging them, or you may feel you are being judged. Perhaps the verse most taken out of context and misapplied is Matthew 7:1, "Judge not, that you be not judged." Sometimes we **must** judge another's actions. Misunderstandings clear up when you read further and in context with other passages of Scripture.

Judge not, that you be not judged. For with the judgment you pronounce you will be judged, and with the measure you use it will be measured to you. Why do you see the speck that is in your brother's eye, but do not notice the log that is in your own eye? Or how can you say to your brother, "Let me take the speck out of your eye," when there is the log in your own eye? You hypocrite, first take the log out of your own eye, and then you will see clearly to take the speck out of your brother's eye. Do not give dogs what is holy, and do not throw your pearls before pigs, lest they trample them underfoot and turn to attack you. … Beware of false prophets, who come to you in sheep's clothing but inwardly are ravenous wolves. (Matthew 7:1 – 6, 15)

How will you recognize the "wolves," "dogs," and "pigs" if you do not judge? When someone is in sin or harming you, **it is perfectly acceptable to judge their actions**. However, when you look at another through the lens of your strongholds, you cannot make a righteous judgment. **First, you must examine your own heart** to discover the truth.

- Did you "take the log out of your eye" by examining your own heart and motives?
- Take an honest look from the other person's perspective. Are they right?
- Is this a situation in which you should show understanding and grace?
- Does your perspective of the conflict seem out of character for the other person?
- Is this an ongoing issue or a simple mistake you can overlook? Not every situation requires confrontation.

Right Judgment

Sometimes we **should** judge, and we **can** discern good and evil. However, right judgment of another's actions requires maturity in Christ.

- You must use discernment to judge righteously; do not base your judgement on appearances.
- You may judge a person's actions as right or wrong by God's standards.
- You are to judge those in the church and purge evil people from your inner circles.
- God judges those outside the church.

And his delight shall be in the fear of the Lord. He shall not judge by what his eyes see, or decide disputes by what his ears hear. (Isaiah 11:3)

I wrote to you in my letter not to associate with sexually immoral people—not at all meaning the sexually immoral of this world, or the greedy and swindlers, or idolaters, since then you would need to go out of the world. But now I am writing to you <u>not to associate</u> with anyone who bears <u>the name of brother</u> if he is guilty of sexual immorality or greed, or is an idolater, reviler, drunkard, or swindler—not even to eat with such a one. For what have I to do with judging outsiders? <u>Is it not those inside the church whom you are to judge</u>? God judges those outside. "<u>Purge the evil person from among you</u>." (1 Corinthians 5:9 – 13)

For everyone who lives on milk is unskilled in the word of righteousness, since he is a child. But solid food <u>is for the mature</u>, for those who have <u>their powers of discernment trained by constant practice</u> to distinguish good from evil. (Hebrews 5:13 – 14)

Do you ever wonder why in one verse are we told to judge some people, and in others we are told not to judge people? The difference is in **how** we judge them.

- We should not pass judgment on unbelievers.
- We must not judge people before checking our own heart (removing the log from our eye).
- Judging wrongly is when we speak evil against a brother (a fellow Christian).
- Right judgment is sincere, impartial, full of mercy, reasonable, gentle, and wise.
- You must not judge a weaker believer for **their lack of faith**.

Therefore you have no excuse, O man, every one of you who judges. For in passing judgment on another you condemn yourself, <u>because you, the judge, practice the very same things</u>. (Romans 2:1)

Do not speak evil against one another, brothers. <u>The one who speaks against a brother or judges his brother, speaks evil</u> against the law and judges the law. But if you judge the law, you are not a doer of the law but a judge. There is only one lawgiver and judge, he who is able to save and to destroy. But who are you to judge your neighbor? (James 4:11 – 12)

But the wisdom from above is first pure, then peaceable, gentle, open to reason, full of mercy and good fruits, impartial and sincere. (James 3:17)

As <u>for the one who is weak in faith</u>, welcome him, but <u>not to quarrel over opinions</u>. (Romans 14:1)

Questions to Ponder

48.4) When have you judged another wrongly? Explain.

48.5) Do you tend to pass judgments on others based on what annoys you?

48.6) When have you judged someone for something that you yourself did/do?

48.7) What does it mean to not judge the world? ("For what have I to do with judging outsiders?")

48.8) Do you argue with or judge others if they hold a different opinion? If so, why?

Engage in Conflict

Scripture tells us to reconcile **with the one who offended** us **and** with **those we have offended**. It is our responsibility to put forth genuine effort to resolve the issue, **regardless of who was at fault**. Our pride and anger often demand that a person come to us for resolution, but this is not God's way. We must take responsibility and resolve the issue in a timely manner. The longer a matter goes unresolved, the more difficult it is to resolve. The longer questions and misconceptions go unanswered, the more opportunity for vain imaginations to make an offense seem worse than it was.

Bearing with one another and, if one has a complaint against another, forgiving each other; as the Lord has forgiven you, so you also must forgive.
(Colossians 3:13)

Be angry and do not sin; do not let the sun go down on your anger,
and give no opportunity to the devil. (Ephesians 4:26 – 27)

When the Issue Is Against You

If you know someone holds an offense against you, examine your heart and see if you are in the wrong. Either way, go to the person and hear their heart on the matter. If you are in the wrong, apologize and repent. If you are confident your actions were right, do your best to help them understand the situation. Apologize for misunderstandings and your part in the offense. Do **not apologize or feel guilt** for a problem you did not create. People often project their guilt onto others when emotions are involved. Set feelings aside and focus on the truth of the situation. Put your best effort into resolution; it is the other person's choice to receive or reject what you say.

If possible, so far as it depends on you, live peaceably with all. (Romans 12:18)

Some things to remember when someone has an issue with you:

- Go to the person you harmed or offended. Do not make them come to you.
- Hear the other person out completely and consider what they say before responding.
- Search your heart and the Lord to discover the truth in the situation.
- Offer an honest apology and repent of any wrongdoing.
- Ask for their forgiveness and ask the Lord to forgive you as well.
- Abide by their wishes regarding how to move forward in the relationship. Do not force forgiveness or push for relationship if they, or you, are reluctant.
- Once you did all you can do, leave the rest in God's hands.

So if you are offering your gift at the altar and there remember that your brother has something against you, leave your gift there before the altar and go. First be reconciled to your brother, and then come and offer your gift.
(Matthew 5:23 – 24)

When the Issue Is with Someone Who Hurt You

"If possible, so far as it depends on you, live peaceably with all" (Romans 12:18). This verse still applies when you are harmed. Examine your heart to see how you may have wronged the other person. In most conflicts, **both people** make mistakes. If needed, start the conversation with an apology to set a tone for reconciliation, but **keep your apology genuine** and do not use it to introduce blame.

- A poor apology would be, "I am sorry I hung up on you, but you are so unreasonable."
- A better apology would be, "I am sorry, I hung up on you. I did not handle my emotions well. I am sorry I hurt your feelings."

Some things to remember when handling an offense:

➤ **Understand the situation.** Journal about the situation to get it clear in your mind.

- What was the exact nature of the wrong against me?
- What was my part in it? How do I feel? How did I respond?
- What is the perspective of the others involved? How might they feel? What emotions led each person's response?
- What was the impact on my life? What did the person's actions threaten?
- What is God's truth? Am I believing the report of the enemy?

➤ **Get right with God.**

- Did I handle the situation biblically? Where do I need to repent?
- Is there an error or character defect in myself that I saw reflected in the other person, or that influenced my response?
- Confess your wrongs to God and seek His forgiveness. Stand ready to forgive the other person for their wrongs to you, regardless of the conflict's outcome.

➤ **See the offender through the loving eyes of God.**

- Remember God's grace and mercy in your life. Have compassion for your offender.
- Remember it is God's nature to restore the offender, just as He wants to restore you.
- Ask the Lord to guide you to reconciliation. The purpose of conflict is to restore wholeness in the relationship, **not to prove that you are right**.

➤ **Prepare yourself for conflict.**

- Prepare your heart to seek the best for both the offender and you in love.
- Prepare your ears to listen to their side.
- Prepare your eyes to see the other person's perspective.
- Prepare your hands to extend grace, mercy, and truth.
- Prepare your feet to walk on the path of peace, searching for reconciliation.
- Prepare your mouth to give answers seasoned with meekness, humility, and respect.

➢ **Confront the one who hurt you.**

- o This is a two-way conversation, and the other's feelings and thoughts may differ from yours. Even though you were wronged, it is important to show the offender respect.

- o Tell the other how you were wrong and ask for forgiveness.

- o Seek clarification, and prepare questions you can ask. This will help you stay on track and focus on finding the truth rather than allowing your emotions to guide the discussion.

- o Tell the offender only what you need him to know about how his actions affected you. Do not bring up past, **resolved** offenses to prove your point.

- o Be gentle and consider their feelings while being firm and straightforward.

- o Use non-threatening communication, such as "I" statements. ("I think," "I feel," "I hope," etc.)

- o Discuss what each person needs to resolve the matter.

➢ **Restoration**

- o If the person listens to you and you both believe the matter is resolved, let the offender know you forgive them and do not continue rehashing the offense.

- o Pray with them and be ready to help the offender overcome his or her transgression.

When the Offender Does Not Listen

What do you do when you try your best to resolve a matter, but the offender refuses to listen?

> *If your brother sins against you, go and tell him his fault, between you and him alone. If he listens to you, you have gained your brother. But if he does not listen, take one or two others along with you, that every charge may be established by the evidence of two or three witnesses. If he refuses to listen to them, tell it to the church. And if he refuses to listen even to the church, let him be to you as a Gentile and a tax collector.*
> *(Matthew 18:15 – 17)*

Take one or two others to bear witness

After attempting resolution with the person one on one, it is okay to take others with you to confront the problem. The implication in this verse in Matthew 18 is **to bring objective people** whose goals are **restoration**, who seek the best interests of both parties, listen with impartiality, and are willing to extend grace and mercy. This verse is not an excuse to **gather allies** that will gang up on the offender and fight your point.

Take it before the church

This is how you handle conflict **with believers**. Obviously, it is not appropriate to drag a non-believer before your church elders to show how they are wrong. How can you hold a non-believer to Christian standards? When an issue with a non-believer cannot be resolved, leave it in the Lord's hands and distance yourself to prevent future harm.

Treat the offender like a Gentile

After every attempt has failed and the individual is clearly unrepentant, "let him be to you as a Gentile or tax collector." Paul shows us what this means in his letters to the churches. The one treated as a "Gentile or a tax collector" is separated from the body of believers, treated like a non-believer, and **put on a path toward repentance for his salvation**. This is meant to be done in love; it is not an excuse to shun him or be cruel. You do not "ghost" the offender or treat him like a leper. Make the problem clear and continue to love and pray for him. The separation puts him in the Lord's hands and protects other believers from his sin. God draws the offender in to deal with his heart.

> *If anyone does not obey what we say in this letter, take note of that person, and <u>have nothing to do with him</u>, that he may be ashamed. <u>Do not regard him as an enemy, but warn him as a brother</u>. (2 Thessalonians 3:15)*

> *You are to deliver this man to Satan for the destruction of the flesh, <u>so that his spirit may be saved</u> in the day of the Lord. (1 Corinthians 5:5)*

Restoring the offender

When the offender realizes his wrongs and chooses change, **be quick to restore him**. If the offender's **repentance is genuine**, even if he repeats past mistakes, he will correct them. **He should return to open and loving arms, comfort, forgiveness, rejoicing, and a fresh start.** Reaffirm your love for him. Do not hold his past wrongs against him but give him the opportunity to earn your trust again.

> *For such a one, this punishment by the majority is enough, so you should rather <u>turn to forgive and comfort him</u>, or he may be overwhelmed by excessive sorrow. So I beg you to <u>reaffirm your love for him</u>. (2 Corinthians 2:6 – 8)*

> *As it is, I rejoice, not because you were grieved, but because you were grieved into repenting. For you felt a godly grief, so that you suffered no loss through us. <u>For godly grief produces a repentance that leads to salvation</u> without regret, whereas worldly grief produces death. (2 Corinthians 7:9 – 10)*

<u>Questions to Ponder</u>

48.9) What did you learn you should do differently when a conflict arises?

48.10) Is there a current situation to which you can apply this lesson? Explain.

48.11) Explain the difference between handling conflict with a believer and handling conflict with a non-believer.

48.12) Have you restored someone as described in this lesson? What was the result?

Lesson 49 — Communication

The way we communicate will always reflect either Christ or the world. It is difficult to communicate in God's love when our emotions are out of control. Preconceived ideas about a person can influence the way we communicate with them. People often hear what they expect, rather than the actual words spoken. **The key to effective communication is for each person to honor the other in the way they listen and the words they speak.**

Effective Listening

❖ **Actively Listen** – Active listening honors the one who is speaking. Instead of planning your reply, give your full focus to comprehending the message the other is trying to convey. It is easy to listen from your perspective and assume a person thinks like you. Ask questions to discover the point that **the speaker** wants you to understand. Give the speaker your full attention and maintain eye contact (but do not stare—that is creepy).

> *Know this, my beloved brothers: let every person be quick to hear,*
> *slow to speak, slow to anger. (James 1:19)*

❖ **Avoid Interrupting** – This is easier said than done, especially when you are a quick thinker, or someone is long-winded. Allow the speaker full expression of his or her thought. The person will feel heard, and you will gain a clearer understanding of their message. Sometimes it helps to jot down notes as a reminder of what they said to address it later, allowing your full focus to stay on the one speaking.

> *A fool takes no pleasure in understanding, but only in expressing his opinion.*
> *(Proverbs 18:2)*

> *If one gives an answer before he hears, it is his folly and shame.*
> *(Proverbs 18:13)*

❖ **Avoid Distraction** – Do not allow pets, children, or other environmental factors to draw your attention away from the speaker. If possible, turn off your phone or silence the notifications.

> *For everything there is a season, and a time for every matter under heaven.*
> *(Ecclesiastes 3:1)*

❖ **Keep an Open Mind** – Do not look for what is wrong in another's words, but listen from his perspective. Listen with impartiality. You may learn something new, or it may alert you to a wrong understanding. Wait for the speaker to finish before deciding whether you agree or disagree.

> *The heart of the righteous ponders how to answer, but the mouth of the*
> *wicked pours out evil things. (Proverbs 15:28)*

- ❖ **Speak Truth in Love** – Make sure your words are honest. In love, speak your genuine thoughts and feelings, even if you know the person will disagree with you. Do not avoid speaking truth to spare someone's feelings but speak with gentleness and compassion when sharing a hard truth. Do not make up stories, exaggerate, or leave out important details. If you cannot speak truth, it is best to say nothing.

  Rather, speaking the truth in love, we are to grow up in every way
  into him who is the head, into Christ. (Ephesians 4:15)

  Better is open rebuke than hidden love. Faithful are the wounds of a friend;
  profuse are the kisses of an enemy. (Proverbs 27:5 – 6)

- ❖ **Be Direct** – Do not talk around an issue to avoid answering a question, hoping a person will "read between the lines." Do not give a disingenuous answer. **Being misunderstood contradicts the purpose of communication.** Get straight to the point and give full, clear descriptions, details, and examples to communicate an unmistakable message to the listener.

  The heart of the wise makes his speech judicious and adds persuasiveness to his lips.
  (Proverbs 16:23)

- ❖ **Use Kind Words** – Honor other people with your words, remembering that unkind words can hurt. Your tongue holds the power of life and death. Before you speak, think about how your words may sound to another. Avoid rejection, avoidance, scorn, sarcasm, ridicule, threats, accusing, or blaming. These are cruel, abusive, and ineffective in communication.

  Let your speech always be gracious, seasoned with salt, so that you may
  know how you ought to answer each person. (Colossians 4:6)

  A gentle tongue is a tree of life, but perverseness in it breaks the spirit. (Proverbs 15:4)

  There is one whose rash words are like sword thrusts, but the tongue of the wise brings healing.
  (Proverbs 12:18)

  Whoever belittles his neighbor lacks sense, but a man of understanding remains silent.
  (Proverbs 11:12)

- ❖ **Use "I" Statements** – Use "I" statements every time you are sad, angry, defensive, or need to confront another person about an issue. It is far more effective to focus your speech on yourself than on another. When the word "you" is used to address a problem, it puts the listener on the defensive. No one wants to hear how they are wrong, but they are more open to hearing you say "I think" or "I feel." Instead of saying, "You left dirty dishes in the sink again," say, "I am upset that the dishes were not done." Or, instead of saying, "Why don't you fix this?" say, "It would help me to know your plans about this." Use "I" statements to express thoughts, feelings, concerns, or to share how a behavior affects you. Then state what you need to happen.

A soft answer turns away wrath, but a harsh word stirs up anger. (Proverbs 15:1)

To speak evil of no one, to avoid quarreling, to be gentle, and to show perfect courtesy toward all people. (Titus 3:2)

Body Language

❖ **Your Body Speaks Louder Than Your Words.** Keep open body language as you engage in communication. Assume a listening position, unguarded and engaged. Your face will give you away if you are disingenuous. If your expressions are interested and reflect the other's feelings, the person will trust your words are genuine. **Your body will speak your language** if you are open and honest.

A worthless person, a wicked man, goes about with crooked speech, winks with his eyes, signals with his feet, points with his finger, with perverted heart devises evil, continually sowing discord. (Proverbs 6:12 – 14)

But I discipline my body and keep it under control, lest after preaching to others I myself should be disqualified. (1 Corinthians 9:27)

Questions to Ponder

49.1) Are your listening skills effective? Where can you improve?

49.2) How can you become more attentive while listening? What distracts you from listening?

49.3) Do you interrupt? Are you considering your response while another is talking?

49.4) How open are you to hearing another person's perspective?

49.5) Are your speaking skills effective? Where can you improve?

49.6) How honest is your communication? Do you say what others expect or want to hear? Do you exaggerate or leave out details?

49.7) Is your communication direct and to the point, or do you try to get your message across without saying what is truly on your mind?

49.8) Do you use many details and examples to make sure your messages are clear?

49.9) Are you thoughtful? How often do you use sarcasm, ridicule, threats, accusations, or blame, to respond to another's questions or comments? Do you ignore them?

Effective Communication

Effective communication may be difficult when you or another have a vested interest in the conversation's outcome. **Be intentional about how you communicate.** The following tips can help:

❖ **Observe the Conversation –** Use your emotions to teach you; do not allow them to control you. Prepare your mind to observe the conversation and actions of others without absorbing their negativity. Let their words roll off you. When you focus your mind on observing, it is more difficult to absorb the other person's words as a personal attack.

> *Do not take to heart all the things that people say, lest you hear your servant cursing you.*
> *Your heart knows that many times you yourself have cursed others.*
> *(Ecclesiastes 7:21 – 22)*

❖ **Do not Become Vexed –** Vexation is when we feel worried, annoyed, or frustrated. One of the greatest traps laid by the enemy is to use other people to push our buttons. Once we lose patience and show annoyance or irritation, we lose the conversation. There is an old saying that you catch more flies with honey than with vinegar. You may not want to catch flies, but this old saying still rings true. When your responses become grumpy or bitter people stop listening. On the other hand, it is impossible to escalate a conflict with someone who always replies sweetly and refuses to be baited into a heated quarrel. Gentle kindness and patience will serve you well. Do not become discouraged when you mess up. Strong emotions make it difficult to respond in love. Keep trying. It will get easier.

> *The vexation of a fool is known at once, but the prudent ignores an insult. (Proverbs 12:16)*

> *With patience a ruler may be persuaded, and a soft tongue will break a bone. (Proverbs 25:15)*

❖ **Be Discerning –** Always seek the Lord's wisdom when communicating with another. Listen for subtle manipulations and falsehoods but respond with kindness. Your integrity is more important than making sure they understand your emotional state. Redirect conversation back to the truth. Use wisdom when deciding what you share and how you speak.

> *The wise of heart is called discerning, and sweetness of speech increases persuasiveness.*
> *(Proverbs 16:21)*

❖ **Respond, Don't React –** Respond to the situation; do not react to it. We **react** in emotion; we plan **responses**. Reactions further turmoil while responses will guide you through the problem. Once your handling of a situation becomes unreasonable, intense emotions overshadow everything you say. Plan a calm, reasoned response.

> *Whoever is slow to anger has great understanding, but he who has a hasty temper exalts folly.*
> *(Proverbs 14:29)*

Planned Communication

When approaching a conflict or difficult conversation, you need a good grasp on what you are thinking and why. When something causes a powerful emotion, do not storm out to confront the person. Instead, make a plan to communicate. Having a plan makes a favorable outcome more likely.

Before communicating

- ❖ **Allow Plenty of Time –** Plan to engage in a serious conversation when neither party feels stress and there is plenty of time available. Do not force or rush a conversation.

- ❖ **Identify Your Emotions and Their Causes –** Know what you feel and why you feel it. Often, the easiest answer is not the only answer. Repeat the question "Why else do I feel this way?" until you can no longer answer. This helps you see a bigger picture of the situation and may help you determine an appropriate course of action.

    - ○ **Example:** I feel angry about_____. I also feel angry about _____. I also feel angry about_____. (Repeat for all emotions: fear, sadness, etc.)

- ❖ **Review the Elements of Effective Speaking and Listening in This Lesson –** It takes a lot of practice to learn alternative methods of communication. Practice prepares you for more challenging conversations.

During communication

- ❖ **Encourage Successful Communication –** You may have excellent communication skills, but that does not mean that the one you are conversing with does. You can, however, direct the conversation to improve communication.

- ❖ **Do Not Overwhelm the Listener –** State clear and precise points using "I" statements. Only offer **one point on one issue** at a time. If you rattle off twenty points at once, it is impossible for the listener to address them all. When confronted with many issues, people often focus on the one they are most comfortable addressing. If you are a listener in this scenario, ask the speaker to return to their first point and deal with issues one by one. They will probably return to the point they consider most important to address.

- ❖ **Ask the Listener to Repeat Your Point –** Many times, conversations go wrong because the listener is not actively listening. Having the listener repeat what you said is a simple way to make sure they clearly understood you.

    - ○ **Example:** "Can you tell me what I said in your own words, so I know you understand me?"

- ❖ **Move on to the Next Point** – After you are certain the other person understands you, move on to the next point. Do not engage in a discussion on each point until you finish speaking, and do not allow the conversation to veer toward a new issue. Ask the listener to hear you out before responding. You may suggest they take notes on something they wish to address after you finish. If they refuse to hear you out, end the conversation until they are ready to listen.

- ❖ **Hear the Other Side** – After you have finished expressing every point, give the listener the same opportunity to respond. Ask them also to state one point at a time and repeat each point back to them: "I heard you say that_____." **Show them the same respect you demand for yourself.** Do not interrupt or cut them off, and make sure you comprehend their message.

After communicating

- ❖ **Make Your Decision** – Once everyone has expressed their thoughts and feelings, end the conversation: "I will consider/pray about what you said." Refuse to **offer or hint** to an answer until you have an opportunity to consider it. Do not allow yourself to be rushed. **Give answers like**, "I understand what you are saying" or "I understand how you feel". **Do not give answers like**, "You may be right" or "Maybe later" or "I think I can _____." These kinds of answers create an opening to be manipulated into making a snap decision. Only give an answer after reflecting and praying about it away from the conversation.

- ❖ **Tell the Other Person Your Decision** – Once you decide about the conversation, tell the other person the truth. Discuss the points on which you agree **and** disagree with them. If the conversation led to a choice, tell them your decision.

A Model to Approach a Difficult Conversation

Use the following model to start a tough conversation. This model will help you approach the person in a loving and non-threatening way.

- ❖ **I know/believe that you** _____. Explain your understanding of the other person's perspective—what you believe they expect, feel, think, or are doing, and why. This helps assure the person of your effort to understand them. It may also clarify the cause of a misunderstanding from the start.

- ❖ **I have been trying to**_____. What are you doing to abide by their wishes, respect their feelings, or correct the situation?

- ❖ **I feel**_____**when** _____. What is the issue you want to discuss?

- ❖ **I would like to see**_____. How do you see the issue resolving?

I tell you, on the day of judgment people will give account for every careless word they speak. For by your words you will be justified, and by your words you will be condemned. (Matthew 12:36 – 37)

Set a guard, O Lord, over my mouth; keep watch over the door of my lips! (Psalm 141:3)

Even a fool who keeps silent is considered wise; when he closes his lips, he is deemed intelligent. (Proverbs 17:28)

Questions to Ponder

49.10) Practice effective listening and effective speaking this week. Write about three times you used these skills and the result of using them.

49.11) Use the planned communication skills and model to have a difficult conversation. When it is finished, reflect: What was the result? Did you find it easy to use?

49.12) Ask your coach to practice these techniques with you.

Chapter Nineteen

Keep Growing
& Move

Lesson 50 — Make Your Recovery Grow

Just when you think you know God, He reveals more. If you spent your lifetime studying God's Word, you would never come close to understanding all God's attributes.

If anyone imagines that he knows something, he does not yet know as he ought to know.
(1 Corinthians 8:2)

There is always a deeper level of relationship and spiritual growth to attain. Do not think you have arrived. The Lord continues to raise you from one level of glory to the next. It only gets better! **Here, your purpose is found in the journey, not the destination.** God sealed the destination the day you gave your life over to Christ. Hold fast to the truths you know but continue to press on to greater things that lie ahead. In this life, it is the journey that matters.

Not that I have already obtained it [this goal of being Christlike] or have already been made perfect, but I actively press on so that I may take hold of that [perfection] for which Christ Jesus took hold of me and made me His own. Brothers and sisters, I do not consider that I have made it my own yet; but one thing I do: forgetting what lies behind and reaching forward to what lies ahead, I press on toward the goal to win the [heavenly] prize of the upward call of God in Christ Jesus. All of us who are mature [pursuing spiritual perfection] should have this attitude. And if in any respect you have a different attitude, that too God will make clear to you. Only let us stay true to what we have already attained. (Philippians 3:12-16 (AMP))

And we all, with unveiled face, beholding the glory of the Lord, are being transformed into the same image from one degree of glory to another. For this comes from the Lord who is the Spirit. (2 Corinthians 3:18)

The rest of your *Rebuilt* lessons will focus on ways to maintain the progress you have made, deal with additional issues as they arise, build healthy habits, and continue to grow ever closer to the Lord. Moving forward requires stepping into a new level of relationship with the Lord to allow His work to grow deeper in your heart.

Questions to Ponder

50.1) **Is there anything stopping you from giving your all to Christ? Explain.**

50.2) **What do you think is the difference between <u>living for</u> Christ and <u>abiding in</u> Him?**

50.3) **What would your life look like if you began living from Him?**

Stop Living for Christ, and Begin Living from Him

If you were asked how you live for Christ, what would you say? You read your Bible, serve your neighbors, serve your church? Are you a prayer warrior? These are important activities for a believer, but if you are not abiding in Christ; they are mere works of your flesh.

Jesus requires more; He requires that we abide in Him. To abide is to remain or continue in Him, to live or dwell in Him. Scripture says we are to lose our lives to save them. Our lives do not belong to us; rather, God bought us for a price. Do you understand the depth of what this means? **The cost of following Christ is giving up your life and living from His.**

For although there may be so-called gods in heaven or on earth—as indeed there are many "gods" and many "lords"— yet for us there is one God, the Father, <u>from whom are all things and for whom we exist</u>, and one Lord, Jesus Christ, through <u>whom are all things and through whom we exist</u>. (1 Corinthians 8:5 – 6)

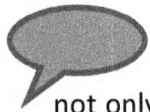

> "Therefore, you must put Him first and then let everything flow from that. Let everything begin with Him and flow forth from Him. That's the secret of life. To not only live for Him, but to live your life from Him, to live from His living, to move from His moving, to act from His actions, to feel from His heart, to be from His being, and to become who you are from who He is ... I am."
>
> Jonathan Cahn, *The Book of Mysteries* (Lake Mary, FL: Frontline, 2016). Used with permission.

God created you unique. His command to give up your life does not suggest giving up the specific traits that make you, <u>you</u>. Instead, it means to submit all of who you are to Christ's will and authority. When you are "all in," you can claim with Paul, "It is no longer I who live but Christ in me" (Galatians 2:20). This is the place where you stop living from your flesh.

The name of God is literally "I AM." His very breath formed everything; all that exists came from his being. **He is our source, which gives us life and sustains us.** Without Christ we are a dying mound of flesh trying to find life in artificial sources, such as our job, friends, success, wealth, family, and even our morals. These are false gods and idols that **give us a false sense of living** but cannot truly give us abundant life.

*I have been crucified with Christ. It is no longer I who live, but Christ who lives in me.
And the life I now live in the flesh I live by faith in the Son of God, who loved me and gave himself for me. (Galatians 2:20)*

Our source must change. **When the world is our source, we live from our need, but when God is our source, we live from Christ's abundance.** Let the essence of who you are, your thoughts, actions, and desires, flow from Him. Allow your "I am" to flow from the "I AM."

To abide in Christ and allow him to abide in you is, in effect, **becoming one with God.** The old corrupt nature no longer has room to exist. As you rise to life in Christ, every surrendered part of you takes on His likeness. Your life becomes Jesus' hands and feet to a lost world. Every word you speak and every thought in your mind is birthed by His wisdom, and He guides each step of your feet.

You would not intentionally remove a limb, pluck out an eyeball, or cut out a healthy organ. **God is part of you, and you are part of Him.** Trying to move without Him would be little different from trying to run a marathon without your legs. Living life **for** God instead of **from** Him is like running a race with artificial limbs. A prosthetic limb can help you get your life back after a devastating injury, but you will never be fully connected to it.

Our sin caused a handicap, which prevents us from living the way God first designed us to live. **In our flesh, we seek artificial gods** to fill this missing part of us. As **believers, we may rely on our religious works** and our understanding, yet we can only become whole by **becoming one with God. He is the missing piece** of our being, which makes us complete.

But he who is joined to the Lord becomes one spirit with him. (1 Corinthians 6:17)

If then you have been raised with Christ, seek the things that are above, where Christ is, seated at the right hand of God. Set your minds on things that are above, not on things that are on earth. For you have died, and your life is hidden with Christ in God. When Christ who is your life appears, then you also will appear with him in glory. (Colossians 3:1 – 4)

Questions to Ponder

50.4) Considering what you have just read, how would you define living *from* Christ?

50.5) How will this look in your life?

Put on the Blinders!

If you have ever witnessed a crime or accident, you know each person's story is different. This does not mean that one person is lying, and another is speaking truth. It is a matter of perspective. Each witness has a distinct vantage point, and as a result, each narrative of the same event varies. None of the witnesses see the complete picture; they can only speak to what each personally saw. Their testimonies are like puzzle pieces. The investigator attempts to fit all the pieces together to form a big picture and discern the truth.

Your eyes are your witnesses, taking in information about current circumstances. **Your mind is the investigator**, making assumptions based on what your eyes perceive, but these are often flawed assumptions. Your witnesses only see from the narrow perspective that revolves around you, filtered through desires, preconceived ideas, worldview, and experiences. **God, however, sees the big picture we cannot comprehend.** He sees details of the heart, which no person can witness. Abiding in Christ allows **a new understanding** from God's perspective, **with healthy eyes** focused on the eternal.

That the God of our Lord Jesus Christ, the Father of glory, may give you the Spirit of wisdom and of revelation in the knowledge of him, having the eyes of your hearts enlightened, that you may know what is the hope to which he has called you, what are the riches of his glorious inheritance in the saints. (Ephesians 1:17 – 18)

The eye is the lamp of the body. So, if your eye is healthy, your whole body will be full of light. (Matthew 6:22)

Discover a God Perspective

The Lord can open the eyes of your heart to new revelation and understanding. It is far easier to seek His truth in times devoted to worship, prayer, and study. When finances, people, and situations become overwhelming, or your desires in life conflict with God's, focusing on the eternal can seem like an impossible task.

To walk in God's truth, put blinders on your natural eyes and see with God's perspective. This is something many believers spend their lives unable to grasp because we function in a natural world. Those who grasp it, like the first believers, live abundant lives, walking with God in boldness, confidence, and contentment.

Use the following suggestions to live life with the mind of Christ:

❖ **Stop Trying to Make God Fit Your Life** – Ask to come into the Lord's presence **to walk with Him** through **His** day. Do not try to make God **or His word** fit your life; instead, make your life fit with Scripture and God's plan. Your relationship with the Lord comes first. Do not worry about what others do; focus on what **you** are doing. When He leads your days, He shows you how to live rightly, who to pray for, and who needs help.

❖ **Do Not Stop Moving** –The law of inertia in physics states that something in motion or rest will stay in motion or rest until acted upon by an outside force. This principle can be applied to your relationship with God. Once you start moving with God, you will continue moving with Him unless an outside force stops you. **Distractions become the force that stops your forward movement with God.** When you are living **for** Christ, any crisis, financial burden, political issue, person, or distraction of the world can take your mind off Him. When your life flows **from** His, directed by His leading, the mundane and difficult tasks of life will not draw you away but bring you closer to Him. Are you giving your attention to worthy things, or are you distracted?

❖ **Rest in God, Not in the World** –It is easy to turn your attention off the Lord to just "live your life." **To be one with God means we can't take a break from Him.** Remember, He bought you for a price; it is not **your** life you are living, but His. He is part of you, and you are part of Him. To claim that you require a break from God is like demanding a break from your right arm.

❖ **How You Rest Matters** –We often confuse entertainment with rest. Have you ever come home from vacation exhausted? Your break **left you entertained, but not rested**. To rest in the Lord, is taking a break from life's burdens to focus your attention on Jesus. True rest is **not fulfilling a litany of religious duties, but** devoting time to **simply enjoy God**, spending intimate time with Him alone, in His creation, or in fellowship with His people. Play is important too, but not at the expense of resting in the Lord. His rest keeps you moving forward. Mind-numbing pursuits or worldly entertainment are not rest but distractions.

❖ **Do Not Grow Weary of Doing God's Work** – You know you have taken back the control you once gave the Lord when you neglect your walk with Christ. Neglecting prayer, study, or worship is a clue that your rest is laziness. You will remain idle until an **outside force**, such as a trial or crisis, brings you back to the feet of the Lord.

❖ **Stop Taking God for Granted; Take Evil for Granted** – We live in a fallen world, and bad things happen. Evil exists. Take this truth for granted. The expectation that bad things happen focuses our eyes on the Lord's blessings, fixing our thoughts on God and strengthening our faith. When we take God and his goodness for granted, every trial and evil grabs our attention. Troubles seem bigger, and doubt creeps in. We may wonder, "Where is God?" or "Why hasn't God acted?" and our faith wavers.

❖ **Remember, Everything Works for Good** – Our minds create a concept of good and bad to determine how we view a situation. This perspective is often founded on what we like or dislike. This is a worldly perspective. When we have the mind of Christ, we can experience joy in our trials because they work for our perfection and completion. God makes "bad" circumstances benefit us, and He blesses us with "good" gifts. When you encounter hardships, focus on the Lord and how He is using the situation to finish His work in you.

Today Starts a New Journey

Let today begin a new journey with the Lord, one that takes you into a deeper relationship, where you stop living for Christ and start living from Him. No longer think of or address the Lord as if He is separate from you. Live as one entity, working for an eternal purpose greater than this world. This is living in truth. Today, as you continue your journey, **you have a choice**. Do you stay where you are, or jump "all in" with Christ?

**We exist *for* God, but our existence flows *from* Him.
We live from Him and through Him.**

❖ It is not about applying the word to your life but living your life from His word.

❖ It is not making scripture fit your life; it is making your life fit the scripture.

❖ It is not about inviting Him to walk with you through your day, it is about asking to come into His presence and walk with Him through His day.

Questions to Ponder

50.6) What is the main understanding you have taken away from this lesson?

50.7) How will you apply a new perspective as you move forward with God?

50.8) How can you change the way you enter God's presence each day?

50.9) Are you setting your attention on activities that do not benefit God's purpose?

50.10) Have you made a choice to be "all in" with God? If not, why not?

50.11) How have you taken God for granted?

50.12) How can you take evil for granted?

Lesson 51 — Preventing Relapse

Satan's strongholds have fallen and now your only stronghold is the Lord. The enemy's arrows bounce off the shield of your faith. Your adversary once fought hard to keep you away from God. He lost that battle, yet he does not lose graciously. His attacks will continue, but now **his goals have changed**. How do you walk through life without falling into former detrimental thoughts and behaviors?

It is important for you to be aware of the enemy's new strategy. He wants to

- **Make you ineffective** for God's Kingdom

- **Tempt you back** into old strongholds

- **Destroy your confidence** in an area God has gifted you

Paul was no stranger to spiritual warfare. He understood that **we have three enemies fighting against us** as we live out a spiritual life with Christ:

- We wrestle spiritual **powers and principalities** of darkness and evil

- We struggle against the **world** (people and systems against God), which hates God and His people

- We battle our own **flesh**

For we do not wrestle against flesh and blood, but against the rulers, against the authorities, against the cosmic powers over this present darkness, against the spiritual forces of evil in the heavenly places. (Ephesians 6:12)

> Obvious demonic or "supernatural" activity may come about because you have opened a door through occult activity or influences, witchcraft, or other agreement held with the devil. You must break your agreement with the enemy and come into agreement with God so you can rebuke the devil in Jesus' name. This may require prayer and fasting. If you feel you need help with demonic attacks or oppression, consult with your *Rebuilt* coach.

Some people understand "spiritual powers and principalities" as only referring to demonic activity, but often **spiritual authorities are subtle, disguising their attacks in what appears good or right in our eyes**. They ally with our flesh and the world to prevent us from pursuing our calling and advancing the Kingdom of God.

Our spiritual enemy attacks our mind, using our flesh to cause thoughts of rejection, loss, desire, anger, or fear. His purpose is to tempt us away from Christ and our calling and cause bouts of depression, temptation, or anxiety. **However, we do not need the devil to sin or tempt us. Our own sin nature may draw us away if we do not keep it in check** by walking with the Holy Spirit. Spiritual enemies may use people, even well-meaning people, to carry out their assignments. **It is vital that you refuse to be a slave to the opinions of man**, testing everything by the Word of God and seeking His confirmation. Rebuke thoughts and ideas contrary to truth. When we are walking with God, the enemy has no power, and our spirit testifies to the truth. We need not worry.

> *But I say, walk by the Spirit, and you will not gratify the desires of the flesh. For the desires of the flesh are against the Spirit, and the desires of the Spirit are against the flesh, for these are opposed to each other, to keep you from doing the things you want to do. (Galatians 5:16 – 17)*

Paul understood how to walk with the Lord without falling into these traps. He encouraged believers to follow his example, and the example of those who walk as he did with the Lord.

> *Brothers, join in imitating me, and keep your eyes on those who walk according to the example you have in us. (Philippians 3:17)*

There are several key things we can learn from Paul's example. In Philippians 3, Paul defines a pattern for life that we should walk in as believers. As we dig into this chapter, we discover this pattern helps us **avoid relapse and walk in freedom** with God.

1. Choose Your Friends Wisely

> *Look out for the dogs, look out for the evildoers, look out for those who mutilate the flesh. (Philippians 3:2)*

Paul tells us to be careful whom we choose to associate with. It matters. As you continue with life after *Rebuilt*, it may be easy to forget what you have learned. You may feel temptation to restore toxic relationships because you assume you can handle them now. The truth is bad company corrupts; at best it may lead your mind away from the Lord. It is vital to your recovery and future journey with the Lord to make careful decisions regarding the people and influences you allow in your life.

Rebuilt has taught you a great deal about avoiding the influence, control, and manipulation of toxic people, **yet anyone can be detrimental to you if you become a slave to their opinions**. When you desire the approval of any person more than God's approval, even those you love, Scripture says you are undeserving of God. The desire for acceptance moves you to compromise your values, your boldness, and your confidence in the Lord, and it **limits you to another person's will**. Any person's opinion that holds more weight than the Lord's will become the "dogs" in the above verse that stop you from reaching your full potential in God. **You do not need to earn the approval of others or fear offending them by your beliefs and opinions.** Find people who accept you and sharpen you without judgment and condemnation; find people "equally yoked."

> *Whoever loves father or mother more than me is not worthy of me, and whoever loves son or daughter more than me is not worthy of me. (Matthew 10:37)*

> *For am I now seeking the approval of man, or of God? Or am I trying to please man? If I were still trying to please man, I would not be a servant of Christ. (Galatians 1:10)*

And he said to them, "You are those who justify yourselves before men, but God knows your hearts. For what is exalted among men is an abomination in the sight of God." (Luke 16:15)

> ### Questions to Ponder
>
> 51.1) Whom do you value time with more than time with God?
>
> 51.2) Whose opinions do you value over God's?
>
> 51.3) What ways do you care about people's opinions?
>
> 51.4) Do you compromise your behavior to gain approval or your words to please or not offend another?
>
> 51.5) Do you fear people thinking you are wrong? Do you often argue your opinions?

2. Be Confident

For we are the circumcision, who worship by the Spirit of God and glory in Christ Jesus and <u>put no confidence in the flesh</u>. (Philippians 3:3)

Of course, as believers we must worship God, giving glory to Jesus, but this verse speaks to more than whom we worship. **Where we place our confidence matters.**

Place your confidence **in your relationship and identity in Christ, in your ability to hear His voice, and in His sovereignty over the outcome of any situation.** You can be confident because it is not your ability you rely on, but God's. Lack of confidence in God gives the enemy a foothold to condemn, shame, frighten, or deceive you. If your confidence is in God and His truth about you, doubt will not become a stumbling block.

Confidence also produces an excitement and boldness for Christ. Your confidence is your witness. Can you imagine telling someone about your love for Christ without confidence in who He is and in your testimony? Who would believe you?

As you continue to walk with the Lord, the enemy may seek to defeat you with condemnation, claiming you are not enough or a failure. He may turn your attention from God's truth back to the opinions of man, tempting you to fear rejection or ridicule. He plays on fears of loss. He speaks doubt, causing you to wonder if the Lord left or is punishing you because you did not "perform" well enough for Him. Remember, all these ideas are lies from hell.

God's mercy is new each morning. **Failure does not equal the end, but an opportunity for growth.** Which is more valuable and truer, God's or man's opinion? You are loved. God knows what you go through. **Trials are a mere steppingstone to a new level of glory** in Christ. Have confidence, because with God your only limits are His convictions; your **possibilities** are limitless!

When doubt and insecurity plague your mind, remember this truth:
The question is not if you are able, but rather if God can make you able.
And He can!

Confidence is not pride

Beware of pride. The enemy feeds on pride to make you ineffective for the Kingdom. Our confidence must be in God, not the flesh. Do not forget that Christ is the source of your victory and healing. It is tempting to think, "I've got this!" but you have nothing without Him. Do not forsake trusting in God for trusting in your own understanding or ability. Your assurance in the outcome of a situation comes from your confidence in God.

Paul continues in verses 4 – 6 to state why he has more than enough reason to be confident. In his flesh, he was righteous under the law, blameless, from the tribe of Benjamin, a zealous Pharisee. The religious world considered him a successful, prominent man, yet he chose confidence not in himself, but in Christ Jesus. **We must do the same.**

No matter how smart or educated we are, or how much scriptural knowledge we possess, our faith belongs in God, not ourselves. We can do good works and give excellent gifts, but without God in us, all our works are like filthy rags. Stay confident in your identity and ability **in Christ**, because your God makes you able to do amazing things.

> *We have all become like one who is unclean, and <u>all our righteous deeds are like a polluted garment</u>. We all fade like a leaf, and our iniquities, like the wind, take us away. (Isaiah 64:6)*

Questions to Ponder

51.6)   List evidence of your identity in Christ to revisit when your confidence fails. List times you heard the Lord's voice, how He has used you, and times He intervened in situations. List times that God showed up when you messed up.

51.7)   Are you enough, as you are, for God? Why or why not?

51.8)   How confident are you that you can do "all things through Christ"?

51.9)   How do you still struggle with pride?

51.10) In what circumstances do you currently attempt to solve or understand situations in your own power or wisdom?

3. Gratitude and Reflection

> *But whatever gain I had, I counted as loss for the sake of Christ. Indeed, I count everything as loss because of the surpassing worth of knowing Christ Jesus my Lord. For his sake I have suffered the loss of all things and count them as rubbish, in order that I may gain Christ, and be found in him, not having a righteousness of my own that comes from the law, but that which comes through faith in Christ, the righteousness from God that depends on faith.*
> *(Philippians 3:7 – 9)*

After describing his prior success and notable stature, Paul reflects on what he once had, stating it was all loss, garbage, rubbish. **Nothing was worth more than what he gained through relationship with Christ.** Paul experienced shipwreck and isolation, torment, torture, imprisonment, and became a martyr for his beliefs, yet he considered his life to be more fulfilling and of higher value with Christ than without Him.

As you continue walking with the Lord, take time to remember everything have gained. Your journals serve as an altar of remembrance to God's miracles in you. Review them as a reminder of how far the Lord has brought you. **Your journey is the evidence you need** to trust God's work and provision in your life when trials shake your hope and faith.

You may think you can never forget what God has done in your life because it was such an amazing feat to overcome. The Israelites, leaving Egypt, saw some of the greatest acts and miracles of God, yet in the wilderness they complained that they had been better off in captivity. They forgot the miracles they experienced because **their focus shifted from the Lord's provision to their circumstances**. You **do not** want to **return to your Egypt!**

Trust in the Lord's goodness to **avoid the trap of ingratitude** and **remorse over loss**. There is always a loss and a gain. **Pursue the more valuable gain.** This life appears valuable but is perishing and worthless. By holding on to this life and old ways, you lose the promised land. To choose the Lord's ways means losing your old way of life. **The life of the believer is a massive exchange program.**

Jesus was everything. He gave up his prominent position to become nothing, carrying the world's burden and becoming our sin. He did this so we could trade in our lives, void of eternal meaning or significance, for an eternal life with position, purpose, and value. **Jesus exchanged His all for our nothing, so we could exchange our nothing for God's all.** What do we gain? We become a vessel containing the spirit of the living, all-powerful God, empowered with all His authority. **You cannot become something until you become nothing.**

Before Paul encountered Jesus, the Pharisees regarded him as a righteous man, yet in God's eyes he was a murderer. After Paul became a follower of Christ, the role switched. He became righteous in God's eyes, but a criminal from the world's point of view. It is best to be seen as nothing by human standards to become everything possible with the Lord.

Remembrance requires praise. Praise God for every goodness in your life and all He continues to do. Keep your mind and prayers full of thanksgiving for your transformation, your redemption, and your righteousness. **You cannot be miserable with a heart full of gratitude**, nor can you grumble when **your focus** is on your blessings. Praise is vital to your life as a believer. Praise the Lord through your prayers, your worship, and your testimony. It is the way you enter God's presence. **Praise grabs God's attention**. It keeps your focus off yourself and on Him, keeping you humble and joyful in the Lord, thus giving you strength.

Enter his gates with thanksgiving, and his courts with praise!
Give thanks to him; bless his name! (Psalm 100:4)

The Lord is my strength and my shield; in him my heart trusts, and I am helped;
my heart exults, and with my song I give thanks to him.
(Psalm 28:7)

About midnight Paul and Silas were praying and singing hymns to God, and the
prisoners were listening to them, and suddenly there was a great earthquake, so that
the foundations of the prison were shaken. And immediately all the doors were
opened, and everyone's bonds were unfastened.
(Acts 16:25 – 26)

51.11) What have you lost to follow God?

51.12) What have you gained through your relationship with Christ?

51.13) Do you struggle or feel regret or loss for that which you have given up? How?

51.14) Do you believe there is more value in what was gained than what was lost? Why?

51.15) What are you grateful for now? Be specific.

51.16) How do you display your gratitude to God?

4. God Moves in Trial

That I may know him and the power of his resurrection, and may share his sufferings, becoming like him in his death, that by any means possible I may attain the resurrection from the dead. (Philippians 3:10 – 11)

Jesus experienced every pain common to humanity—persecution, rejection, loss, grief, and fear—yet he never abandoned the Father. Your life should reflect Jesus, in every way, including through times of persecution and trial. It is about the journey and your character, not the outcome. **How you handle a problem is more important than the problem.** Remember God's promises to you and view your struggles from the Lord's perspective. A worldly mindset cannot produce unwavering faith.

It is during life's struggles and trials that we may relapse into old ways, yet it is those same trials that increase our faith and enhance our maturity and closeness with the Lord. **How the trial affects you depends on how you perceive it.** Scripture says to have joy in your trials. Think about how God will work the trial for good.

Joy is eternal, found in God regardless of the circumstance. His Word delights your heart. He is your safe place, your constant standard, never changing, never failing. Joy is the promised end of suffering and the key to standing firm when facing hardship, but how do you have joy when your world is falling apart? In Him, every trial becomes a disguised blessing to rejoice in.

Though the fig tree should not blossom, nor fruit be on the vines, the produce of the olive fail and the fields yield no food, the flock be cut off from the fold and there be no herd in the stalls, yet I will rejoice in the Lord; I will take joy in the God of my salvation. (Habakkuk 3:17 – 18)

Count it all joy, my brothers, when you meet trials of various kinds. (James 1:2)

Rejoice in Him! Rejoice in the Lord always; again, I will say, Rejoice. (Philippians 4:4)

In trials, your joy comes from your hope in the Lord. Unlike false hope in a person, desire, or self, which may fail, **this hope does not depend on a certain outcome**. It trusts God's will and character, believing He is right and has control of the result. God is your refuge, protection, and security. Trust Him. It is when we grow weary of waiting and try to take back control that we stumble.

Trials end in God's time, not our time. Do not allow impatience or **seeking a desired outcome** to turn your focus **away from God** and **onto the trial**. Pray constantly, seeking the Lord's truth, guidance, wisdom, and counsel. Search for God's movement in the situation.

May the God of hope fill you with all joy and peace in believing,
so that by the power of the Holy Spirit you may abound in hope. (Romans 15:13)

Rejoice in hope, be patient in tribulation, be constant in prayer. (Romans 12:12)

When our desire is God, He is faithful to give us our desires. If your love and delight are in the Lord, He gives you Himself. **Our desire for a specific result causes worry.** Instead, desire His will to be done. Regardless of how it appears in the moment, you can trust that His outcome is the right answer for every problem. Do not allow troubles in this world to cause you to neglect worship and quiet stillness with the Lord. It is in the secret place, where you sit and enjoy the Lord, that your spirit finds His presence and your joy is full. It is in the Lord that you will find the greatest pleasure, even amid your trials.

Delight yourself in the Lord, and he will give you the desires of your heart. (Psalm 37:4)

You make known to me the path of life; in your presence there is fullness of joy;
at your right hand are pleasures forevermore. (Psalm 16:11)

Questions to Ponder

51.17) What promises from the Lord should you remember during hard times?

51.18) How can you experience joy in trials?

51.19) How would you describe your desire for the Lord? What do you desire more than Him? This may become a stumbling block in the future.

51.20) How do you have hope when things look impossible?

51.21) Whom in your relationship circles can you lean on when you feel impatient?

51.22) Whom can you depend on to discuss and study Scripture? Who will pray for and with you?

5. Move Forward

Brothers, I do not consider that I have made it my own. But one thing I do: forgetting what lies behind and straining forward to what lies ahead, I press on toward the goal for the prize of the upward call of God in Christ Jesus.
(Philippians 3:13 – 14)

Forgetting what lies behind requires keeping your mind set on forward movement. **Put old ways, old thoughts, and old behaviors to rest** and pursue righteousness. Pressing forward in God's calling on your life cannot include regretting your past or dwelling on what you once had in the world. You cannot forget the person you were, **but as your character transforms, looking more like Christ, the old you will become like a stranger**. Christ defines you; the world no longer has claims on your identity. Your life is no longer your own; a new adventure awaits.

Why do people celebrate a new year? It is a marker in time designated for new beginnings, offering opportunities to start fresh and choose differently. Each new year presents a choice. **You may choose to grieve the loss of the passing year or rejoice in the hope and newness of the unknown and unseen future.** You are embarking on such a season in your life. Will you celebrate the possibilities or grieve the loss of what was?

The "what if's" in your thoughts can become your downfall, keeping you stuck in a cycle of emotional turmoil and ineffectiveness. When you try to predict or assume the future, it is like casting a fishing pole to see what bites. What you bait your hook with determines what you will catch. The question "What if I fail?" will set you up for failure. "What if they reject me?" sets you up for rejection. The "what if's" you believe can become self-fulfilling prophecies. This is not the same as New Age positive thinking mantras, by which people believe they have absolute control over what happens to them. But your actions do reflect what you believe, and **what you believe becomes your reality.**

What if you asked different questions? "What if God uses me?" "What if I succeed?" "What if God's Word is true for me?" Your thoughts then become set on success and not failure. You will see alternative possibilities to strive toward, instead of working to avoid scenarios that may not happen. How would your reality change if your self-talk were spoken with confidence as opposed to fear? Fish for victory, not defeat!

Questions to Ponder

51.23) What old thoughts, behaviors, beliefs, or actions keep resurfacing? Choose to replace them with truth. With what truth will you replace them?

51.24) What doubts cause you to ask "what if" questions?

51.25) What new questions can you ask yourself when you begin to doubt?

51.26) Are there other ways that you may be holding on to your past self?

---

6. Keep Growing

> *Not that I have already obtained this or am already perfect, but I press on to make it my own, because Christ Jesus has made me his own. ... Let those of us who are mature think this way, and if in anything you think otherwise, God will reveal that also to you. (Philippians 3:12, 15)*

In these verses, Paul acknowledges he is not perfect, but continues to strive for perfection. We too strive for righteousness and perfection, always growing in the Lord. However, **do not think you have "arrived" or understand everything about God**, even as you mature in your faith. Paul also says that if you become prideful in this, God will reveal the truth.

As the Lord speaks to the church of Ephesus,

But I have this against you, that you have abandoned the love you had at first. Remember therefore from where you have fallen; repent, and do the works you did at first. If not, I will come to you and remove your lampstand from its place, unless you repent.
(Revelation 2:2 – 5)

The church of Ephesus in Revelation seemed to do everything right, but they missed one crucial point. God demanded repentance because they abandoned their love for Him. When our works are no longer done out of Christ's love, but became a religious duty or driven by ambition, they become worthless. **Do not become prideful and forget for whom you work.**

God tells this church to "remember" and "repent." You can think of your journal as a memorial to the mess the Lord has brought you through. The Ephesians church was told to **remember and return to their past works**. They forgot the love and enthusiasm they first had for the Lord when they experienced freedom in Christ. Your journals are not a memorial to your mess, but to the goodness of your God to deliver you. **Continue journaling** your growth in Christ as a record of your freedom. Review your journals often to help remember your love.

It can be easy to fall into the trap of believing you require less study or no longer need to pray before every decision because you now have it all together. You are together because the Lord holds you together and makes you grow. Even as a mentor, you continue learning from the one you disciple. **No matter how much you know, you can always learn from those you lead.**

Continue to seek the wisdom of your coach. After *Rebuilt*, you can still benefit from your coach, even if you are coaching others. Allow your coach to continue being the iron that sharpens you, and you will continue to sharpen him or her. God speaks directly to us, yet He designed us to need one another for support, accountability and direction. In His infinite wisdom, God chose to use people to be His ministers and mouthpiece. He will continue to use your coach in your life.

Once you stop learning and growing, you operate from your own ability. This is the starting place of pride. God will destroy your pride. The more prideful you are, the more you must endure for Him to reveal your flaws. Stay humble. You will not "arrive" in this life. If Paul, who wrote much of the New Testament, did not arrive, what makes you assume you will (or that you have already done so)? Remember this as your journey continues. The future holds greater understanding for you, as the Lord takes you from one level of glory to the next. Never stop learning. Never stop asking questions and seeking more of God.

Questions to Ponder

51.27) How will your journaling change after *Rebuilt*?

51.28) Are there a places in your life where you feel you have "arrived"? List them.

51.29) What possible temptations for pride exist in your life now?

51.30) How do you learn from people who are less spiritually mature than you?

51.31) What would you still like to learn about God?

51.32) Where would you like to grow more?

7. Cling to the Truth

Only let us hold true to what we have attained. (Philippians 3:16)

The relapse for an alcoholic occurs long before he takes a drink. It begins when his thinking first veers away from what he learned in recovery—possibly weeks before his actions confirm the relapse. The same is true for any issue you are overcoming. Relapse always occurs in the mind first. **The battle to prevent relapse begins with the first thought that is contrary to the truth you have attained.**

If it is difficult for you to catch wrong thinking before it becomes a problem, know it does become easier the longer you walk in truth. No lazy or impulsive mind considers consequences. Stay alert to prevent adverse thoughts from gaining power in your mind.

The most common gateways to relapse are

- Pride/control
- Temptation
- Doubt
- Frustration
- Fear
- Loss/trauma
- Fatigue/being overwhelmed
- Impulsive behaviors

When you find yourself faced with any of the above, use the "Stop, Drop, and Roll" exercise from Book One. Immediately take captive any thoughts that contradict, compromise, or conceal the truth and subject those thoughts to God's truth.

Have you ever had a disturbing thought, recognized the lie and dismissed it, just to have the same thought return later? Before you know it, you act as if the thought is true, even though your rational mind knows it is false. Why does this happen? **It is a slow progression from thought to belief.** Positive thinking is not the same as believing truth. The difference involves **a choice**. You must **choose** to believe the truth over the lie. Think of it like flipping on a light switch. When you flip the switch, you are **choosing** to believe God's word and arrest the lie.

There is no other option, God's light switch is either on or off. When false thoughts creep in, **choose** to reject them by turning on the light of God's Word. The goal, of course, is to **always keep the light on**, but it takes a fight of faith to accomplish this.

Everything is a choice:

- ✓ **Depressed?** Choose worship.
- ✓ **Discouraged by others' opinions?** Choose God's truth.
- ✓ **Anxious?** Choose trust.
- ✓ **Feeling not good enough?** Choose grace and mercy.
- ✓ **Angry?** Choose forgiveness.
- ✓ **Feeling proud or like you need to control a situation?** Choose humility.
- ✓ **Grumbling or complaining?** Choose praise and gratitude.
- ✓ **Suffering injustice?** Choose love.

Questions to Ponder

51.33) Which issues in your life have been the most difficult to overcome?

51.34) How do you respond to each of the gateways to relapse mentioned above?

51.35) How quick are you to notice a detrimental thought?

51.36) What truths will take captive your recurring false thoughts?

51.37) Consider ways you may struggle in the future. How can your coach continue to be a support for you?

Lesson 52 — Prepare!

Daily Diligence

The past year has been an intentional movement forward with God, but what happens next week when the daily motivation of this journey ends? Will you return to your old routine?

> *That he [Christ] might sanctify her, having cleansed her by the washing of water with the word, so that he might present the church to himself in splendor, without spot or wrinkle or any such thing, that she might be holy and without blemish. (Ephesians 5:26 – 27)*

> *"Let us rejoice and exult and give him the glory, for the marriage of the Lamb has come, and his Bride has made herself ready; it was granted her to clothe herself with fine linen, bright and pure"—for the fine linen is the righteous deeds of the saints. (Revelation 19:7 – 8)*

You are heading into a season of testing and growth, transforming you into the flawless bride of Christ. Continue with the **same dedication and commitment**. Enter this new season **set apart** for God, seeking to know the Bridegroom more intimately.

The Mindset of Growth

Completing *Rebuilt* is not an end but a beginning. This journey birthed new understanding, introducing God as a Father who raises you up to your ultimate purpose, making you a bride for His Son. Like a toddler, you are learning to walk. You possess the mind of Christ, no longer a mind of flesh or religion. Still, an old stronghold may resurface. You are a spiritual child in a stage of growth. **Reaching maturity in Christ means you grow well, but in this life, you will never stop growing.** How do you grow well? You learn from watching your Father and mimicking Him. You grow because He increases you!

- You do not save yourself. You do not mature yourself, and you cannot fix yourself.
- Your own effort, prayer, study, or work cannot force you to grow in God.
- You grow by knowing the Lord and His character and His ways.
- **You grow through relationship with God.**

Young children grow and learn by watching their parents. As a toddler learning to take steps, you were not thinking about becoming a premier athlete. You did not beat yourself up when you stumbled or fell. You simply stood up and walked again, each step building on the last until your walk became strong. In the end, you learned to run.

Your spiritual walk is like that of the child learning to walk. You cannot learn to walk forward by examining the past or worrying about failures and mistakes. The time for that is over. The purpose of *Rebuilt* was to prepare you to walk forward.

Children spend years watching their parents' behavior and character, and they grow into a portrait of their parents. Like that little child, you must learn by mimicking the actions and character of your Father, observing Him through His Word, His Spirit, and the witness of His people. **As we observe and learn the Lord's character and ways, we transform into the likeness of our heavenly Father.**

When You Stumble or Fall

Maturity in Christ means **growing well and failing well**. Putting the past behind you does not mean old character flaws will never resurface. God removes our deeply ingrained false beliefs one piece at a time, layer by layer. A person's words or a circumstance may trigger a thought which allows jealousy, fear, control, or insecurity to sneak its way back into your heart. Be careful to avoid the trap of doubt if old behaviors, thoughts, and feelings resurface. Instead of dwelling on your failure, search your heart for the problem the Lord is trying to reveal. Bring it to Him and **continue in a new understanding of an old lesson**.

If the Lord brings a new character issue to light, examine its root, uncover the truth, repent, surrender it, and return to God with a clean slate. **Do not fear more pruning.** Like a stumbling toddler, realize the error, get up, and try again. Never forget you nailed your flaws and failures to the cross. Reject the enemy's lies and move on.

It is important to recognize trials and failures are a good thing. Every obstacle teaches a valuable lesson. It is in these moments that our growth is the greatest. Be open to being wrong and reject feelings of insecurity and unworthiness. Instead, ask yourself, **"What is God doing?"** and **"What does this teach me?"**

For the sake of Christ, then, I am content with weaknesses, insults, hardships, persecutions, and calamities. For when I am weak, then I am strong. (2 Corinthians 12:10)

Each morning becomes a new opportunity for a **fresh start**. Failure does not mean you have lost the Lord's favor. When you become disillusioned, keep true to who you are in Christ. Stay content, knowing God works everything for your benefit.

For his anger is but for a moment, and his favor is for a lifetime.
Weeping may tarry for the night, but joy comes with the morning. (Psalm 30:5)

Questions to Ponder

52.1) Consider the "Mindset of Growth." What are the most important points to apply in your walk with the Lord?

52.2) Are there still strongholds and character flaws with which you struggle?

52.3) Which strongholds or character flaws do you feel you have completely overcome?

52.4) How will you think about future problems, failures, or trials?

Vision and Plans

But, as it is written, "What no eye has seen, nor ear heard, nor the heart of man imagined, what God has prepared for those who love him." (1 Corinthians 2:9)

Where do you see your future? Do you have a desire to serve God's Kingdom stirring in your heart? If you seek His direction and guidance, He will lead each step to fulfill that desire. A life submitted to the Lord's will is greater than your expectations and imaginations, and it will translate into an eternal purpose.

Live out your plans in confidence but **stay flexible for God's detours**. When you are rigid, unwilling to bend past your ideas of what should be, you limit the Lord and your possibilities.

Commit your work to the Lord, and your plans will be established. (Proverbs 16:2 – 3)

Discover Your Calling

God calls every person for one main purpose: to know Him and make Him known. Beyond that, everyone also has a unique purpose for their life and gifts that aid this purpose. People often refer to the latter as their calling. God may call you into a specific occupation, role, or ministry, but it is your relationship with Him that paves the way to a more fulfilling life. So how do you find your specific calling? **The simple answer is you don't.** Your calling finds you.

When God calls you into a ministry, He makes it quite clear. He prepares the way forward and readies your heart and character for the challenges ahead. If you try to jump into your calling unprepared, you may fall into pride. People who serve in ministry roles often fail because they get caught up in pride, mistaking their anointing for their own skill and ability. Their pride may lead to other sins, such as sexual or financial sins. **Be careful not to get stuck on a title, ministry, how your role appears, or how quickly it should grow.** Do not overthink it. Walk with the Lord. He will guide you, one step at a time, toward success.

<u>Do not despise these small beginnings</u>, for the LORD rejoices to see the work begin, to see the plumb line in Zerubbabel's hand. (Zechariah 4:10, NLT)

Allow your life to become a living testimony of God. The Lord sets you apart as His ambassador, to represent Him. The world watches you closely with curiosity and skepticism. The words and actions of every believer display a picture of God to them. **If you look like everyone else but claim the gospel message, they see a hypocrite. If you look like Jesus, they see the truth of God in you.**

God often calls people into a ministry that makes use of their talents and gifting. Are you an artist? Your art can glorify God. Jesus does not call everyone to serve in church ministry, but He calls every believer to be a witness and light to a dark world. Your witness is no less valuable in your workplace, home, hobbies, or civic service. Are you a songwriter, a carpenter, a graphic designer, a mechanic? Each of these skills can benefit God's Kingdom and may become your ministry, but **sometimes your calling is completely unrelated to your abilities**.

God's calling on your life may relate to an area where the enemy attacks you most. Satan loves to preempt a move of God. A socially awkward person may become a pastor. A person insecure in their words may become a mouthpiece for God. The teen kicked out of school, unable to graduate, may become a professional author. The bossy know-it-all, ridiculed their entire life, may become a prominent leader. The selfish business executive may give his life to help people in need. **It is in our weaknesses that we find our greatest strengths in God.**

Moses was not seeking to be the deliverer of Israel when God sent him; he was simply curious about a bush that was on fire but did not burn. Moses was not trying to become the Moses we read about in Scripture. He just obeyed God, and God used his life to prepare him for what he was to become. **You do not need all the answers.** The important thing is to keep growing in the Lord.

It may be awkward at first to walk in your true calling, but soon the calling will feel like home. As God calls you into your purpose and equips you for success, you will discover there is nothing in the world you would rather do. **Stay open-minded to his plans.**

It can be tempting to **create a calling** for yourself **or usurp another person's calling** as your own. The book of Numbers tells the story of Korah, a Levite during the time of Moses and Aaron. God appointed the Levites for all the tabernacle service, but this honor did not satisfy Korah. He was envious of Aaron, chosen as the high priest. Korah's jealousy and envy of a calling that did not belong to him brought a rebellion that ended his ministry and his life.

How can you receive a calling that God has set aside for another? If you are seeking to be an evangelist but God called you to be a youth minister, you may function as an evangelist but fail to prosper in that role. When you stop pursuing a blessing that belongs to another and pursue your true purpose, you will receive the Lord's full blessings. **You cannot become who God created you to be if you are acting like someone you are not.**

Appoint Your Days

So teach us to number our days, that we may get a heart of wisdom. (Psalm 90:12)

This verse speaks about using our time productively because our days on earth are few. But this does **not** imply that you should become busier. Rather, it speaks to how you spend time. The word for numbering in Hebrew is *manah*. It means to appoint, reckon, or count. Numbering your days speaks to appointing or **purposing** each day for the Lord. Your life set apart for the Lord means **your time belongs to Him**. The reward is a heart of wisdom.

Each day offers new opportunity and purpose. **How you start off your morning sets the tone for your day.** It can transform your perspective and prepare your heart for whatever comes. Before your feet hit the floor, give the Lord your attention, your day, your prayers, and worship. **Consecrate each day to the Lord, dedicating it for His purposes.**

Numbering your days is more than making plans; it is making every moment of every day purposely dedicated to Him. **Each moment presents a choice** to do or not do something. **Every choice follows one of two paths**: to walk God's path or follow the ways of the world. Let the Lord direct your every thought, word, and step. He opens doors and exposes wrong choices.

But seek first the kingdom of God and his righteousness, and all these things will be added to you. (Matthew 6:33)

Be careful how you choose to spend your time and consider for whom you are spending it. The world distracts you with **worthless pursuits** that steal your time and attention. Anything that indulges this world and its values is worthless. Limit worthless pursuits. A **worthwhile pursuit** progresses your relationship with God and your calling or purpose. Ask yourself, "Does this benefit the purpose God gave me?"

You adulterous people! Do you not know that friendship with the world is enmity with God? Therefore whoever wishes to be <u>a friend of the world makes himself an enemy of God</u>. (James 4:4)

Therefore, my beloved brothers, <u>be steadfast, immovable, always abounding in the work of the Lord</u>, knowing that in the Lord your labor is not in vain. (1 Corinthians 15:58)

Whoever works his land will have plenty of bread, but
he who follows worthless pursuits lacks sense. (Proverbs 12:11)

Which activities in your normal day are worthwhile pursuits? Fun activities with your children or spouse may appear frivolous but may also enhance those relationships. However, if you are seeking fun to gratify the flesh with entertainment, your priorities could be wrong. Pray and use discernment to determine if your pursuits are in line with God's will.

Whatever you do, work at it with your whole being, for the Lord and not for men.
(Colossians 3:23, BSB)

Questions to Ponder

52.5)   What does it mean to prepare your days to walk with the Lord?

52.6)   How will setting apart your day change the choices you make throughout the day?

52.7)   Considering the vision, calling, and purpose the Lord has shown you for your life, what tasks would you consider *worthwhile* pursuits?

52.8)   Examine your normal activities for the day. Which are *worthless* pursuits?

52.9)   What activities are *ignoble*, neither worthwhile nor worthless? (This includes necessary, mundane tasks.)

52.10) Examine your motives for Christian activities (i.e., prayer, worship, serving, and studying). Are you seeking to earn the Lord's approval, or to know Him more?

Negotiables and Non-negotiables

It is never easy to appoint your days for God while balancing life's obligations. Are you a person who schedules every minute of your day? Or is routine difficult for you? Does an incomplete to-do list discourage you? If allowing the Lord to guide your day seems impossible under the burden and demands of life, **it is time to reexamine your tasks**.

Make two lists

Flexibility allows time for God's unexpected plans and divine appointments, yet there are some tasks you should never neglect. List your **non-negotiable** tasks, things you must do regardless of what happens. This is a very brief list that only includes "worthwhile pursuits." For a believer, this list **will include** personal time with God, prayer, worship, studying Scripture, and journaling. You may have other commitments that you consider non-negotiable, such as specific special moments with your family, praying with your children before bed, or even a family game night.   Your non-negotiable list **does not include** meetings, routines, or appointments on your calendar. You may reschedule these if something or someone else needs your time. Therefore, although they may be a high priority, they *are* negotiable and not mandatory.

Everything **not** on this list is **negotiable**, including meetings, phone calls, social media, videos or television, appointments, your worthless pursuits, and sometimes even baths and sleep. **Negotiable tasks are flexible.** Think differently about what you must do. Some negotiables may seem mandatory, such as meal preparation. Of course, you must eat, but **when** you eat may be flexible, or you can plan a simple dinner in a pinch. List your negotiable daily tasks and activities.

Finally, **prioritize the negotiable list**. Think of this list as your daily "to-do" list. Sort this list by items most important to complete. Your non-negotiable and negotiable lists will rarely change, but you may need to review your priorities daily. A low priority one day may become a foremost priority the next day as your situation changes.

Use your lists

The goal of a non-negotiable list is to make you **less busy**. The important, life-altering tasks will take priority over every other task. After finishing the non-negotiables, complete any tasks on your negotiable list in your remaining time. **Negotiables never replace non-negotiables** and are always subject to the Lord's plans for your day. To live this way **lightens your schedule for unexpected situations** that require your attention.

It is important not to skimp on non-negotiables to allow for negotiable tasks. Your non-negotiables will become routine or obligatory if your schedule restricts their available time so you can fit in all your negotiable tasks. Remember, the Lord's timing is perfect. You truly do not need to accomplish everything you think you do.

If, for example, you limit your quiet time with the Lord to a specific time frame, your focus will divert to the time and obligation of your prayer, rather than the prayer itself. How much revelation can you receive when you cut short your time studying the Word? Is it possible to determine how much time you should worship God, how long you speak to Him, or the time He has available to speak to you? Try not to restrict God's time. When seeking the Lord becomes routine, like making an appointment with the Lord, **it is like checking off a religious duty instead of enjoying a relationship.**

I Can't Do That!

You may believe you are too busy to give God unlimited time, but this is not true. Martin Luther once said, "If I fail to spend two hours in prayer each morning, the devil gets the victory through the day." The enemy would distract, interrupt, and distort him from his purpose. He also said, "I have so much to do that I shall spend the first three hours in prayer." The Lord focused his mind and established his plans for the day. Martin Luther knew he needed to give the Lord time first to accomplish all he needed. He is not alone. Many prominent (and busy) people claim they pray for hours each morning to be productive.

Sometimes your mind will fight against the non-negotiables. Even when you struggle, you can pray, worship, or read Scripture. Often when we do not "feel like it," we actually need it most. Be obedient. **Half the battle is beginning**, and the "feeling like it" will come.

> ### Questions to Ponder
> **52.11) Create a list of the non-negotiables in your life. Keep this list minimal. Many things that are important to you are still negotiable.**

52.12) Create a list of negotiable activities in your normal day. This should be a generic list. (Instead of listing every appointment, you could simply list the type of appointment, such as work meetings, doctor appointments, *Rebuilt* meetings, church functions, etc.)

52.13) From your negotiable list, choose 3 items that are the highest priority. (When choosing, think, "If I cannot do anything else today, I will do this.")

52.14) Bring your lists to the Lord. Seek His heart about them. Do you feel there is something God wants you to add or remove from the non-negotiable list? Is there anything He wants you to make a higher priority?

Obligation and Distraction

One of the hardest things to surrender may be your schedule, especially if you have a family and children. **We often treat unnecessary things like requirements.** God knows the tasks we should and should not do. Give Him your days because His timing is perfect, and His plan is flawless.

God is not in a hurry; why are you? His plan will keep you busy, but His leading does not make you feel driven. The Lord may put an urgency in your heart, but if you seem rushed or pressured, it is likely your flesh, other people, or the enemy, not God.

People often put their needs or expectations on your days. Intentionally or not, people take advantage and disrespect your time. **The ability to say "No" is the most important lesson you can learn.** You should not do something simply because you can. People's expectations must take second place to your non-negotiables and to the Lord. Plenty of time is available for needed tasks, but not always for expected tasks. **Your responsibility is to God's checklist**, not to the desires of family, friends, and neighbors. Your non-negotiables must take precedence over everything else, keeping you flexible to minister where the Lord sends you. **Listen for the Lord to direct you to whom you should help and how.**

To allow pressure, demands, phone calls, social media, distractions, or other confusion to rob you of those most important things **will** cause you to lose focus. Take your negotiable tasks to the Lord and let His timing prevail. A delay rarely becomes a serious problem, although people may make it seem that way.

1. **Slow down.** God is not in a hurry. His plans never fail.

2. **Do not limit God's time.** Nothing is more important than your relationship with Him.

3. **Trust God.** It is okay if something does not get done. God knows your responsibilities, commitments, and desires. All things happen in God's perfect timing.

4. **Let God lead.** We can easily get distracted from the tasks we should do.

52.15) What things or activities distract you from what you should do?

52.16) Which people in your life distract you from what you should do?

52.17) To whom do you have difficulty saying "No"?

52.18) Do you feel pressured, hurried, or driven? What or who causes these feelings?

52.19) How will you slow down?

Test Everything

Test everything; hold fast what is good. Abstain from every form of evil.
(1 Thessalonians 5:21 – 22)

Testing everything is more than testing spirits; it is testing your words and deeds and the words and deeds of others. Were the messages you heard today founded on truth? Stay true to what the Lord has shown you. Do not waver and do not doubt.

Check your heart throughout the day and in the evening. Where did you doubt? What temptations did you have? How did you handle mistakes? How did you do **well**? What frivolous activities did you engage in? Did you make progress? Can you do better?

But if we judged ourselves truly, we would not be judged. But when we are judged by the Lord, we are disciplined so that we may not be condemned along with the world.
(1 Corinthians 11:31)

Judge yourself honestly and you will not be judged. We are tested in our weakness. Guard your mind at all costs and keep your eyes focused on the Lord. Be honest with yourself about the true condition of your heart. **Denial is Satan's best friend.** It is when we are too afraid or ashamed to admit our faults that the enemy sets us up for disaster. When we are honest about our weakness, the Lord works in it and transforms it into our greatest strength.

When you examine the truth of your heart and honestly see your sin, you can give it to the Lord. Avoiding issues keeps you buried under hidden shame. Admitting mistakes allows you to correct them, seek forgiveness, and keep going. It is good to experience the gravity of your wrongs. Without remorse, you will continue in or return to the sin. **Likewise, it is good to learn from your errors, forgive yourself, and put it behind you.** God renews us after we fall. **Why would you continue punishing yourself?**

Questions to Ponder

52.20) How well do you recognize your failings and sin?

52.21) Tell how the Lord has used past failures for your benefit.

52.22) Do you feel you must punish yourself or continue dwelling on past wrongs? Why?

(Continue to the Daily Heart Check.)

Daily Heart Check

A good way to judge yourself honestly is with a daily heart check. Contemplate your day each evening as you journal. Search your heart for wrongs you have done and ways you have walked righteously. Keep your eyes on the Lord regardless of what is happening around you. Continue having the mind of Christ, your love and thoughts unified with the Lord.

Purge me with hyssop, and I shall be clean; wash me, and I shall be whiter than snow. Let me hear joy and gladness; let the bones that you have broken rejoice. Hide your face from my sins and blot out all my iniquities. Create in me a clean heart, O God, and renew a right spirit within me. (Psalm 51:8)

So if there is any encouragement in Christ, any comfort from love, any participation in the Spirit, any affection and sympathy, complete my joy by being of the same mind, having the same love, being in full accord and of one mind. (Philippians 2:1 – 2)

1. **In the morning** – Begin your day by consecrating it for the Lord's purposes. Pray, worship, and study.

2. **Throughout the day** – Seek the Lord every moment and choose His ways in each decision. Guard your mind to keep the mind of Christ.

3. **In the evening** – Journal about your day and perform a short heart check. Thank the Lord for your blessings and the work he is doing in your heart through your trials.

The following questions may help you evaluate your day and check your heart.

- Was there conflict today? Did I ignore it or address it? What in my heart may have led me to see this issue incorrectly?

- In what situations did I fail today? In what ways did I place confidence in my ability apart from the Lord?

- How did I do well today? Where did I have confidence in God's work through me?

- Am I thankful for something I used to take for granted?

- How was I distracted? Are distractions taking from more important things? How can I solve this issue?

- Has something occurred today that brought forth regret, discontent, or ingratitude?

- Am I worried? Where is the hope in this situation?

- Did I have patience and seek the Lord as I walked through my day?

- How did I grow in the Lord today?

- Did I have pride today, or did I try to control a circumstance? Did I doubt God?

- Was I tempted today?

- Did I feel (and how did I handle) fear, insecurity, frustration, fatigue, or being overwhelmed?

- Is a major issue happening in my life right now? Am I trusting God for the outcome? Am I seeking the Lord for wisdom and giving Him control?

- What is God showing and teaching through my trials today? Am I trusting Him in the trials?

Your Final Assignment

The most important part of your recovery is writing and sharing your testimony. Your testimony is the reality of God's goodness, shown through your personal story. Sharing truth learned, and the experience of being set free by that truth, draws others to Christ.

In the Scripture stories, when people experienced God's miraculous work, they built an altar to the Lord. Noah came off the ark and built an altar. God gave land to Abraham, and he built an altar. God gave Isaac land with a promise to multiply his descendants, and Isaac built an altar. **Scripture contains many such examples of altars and memorials to the Lord.**

God knows people's memories are short. Memorials help His people remember His goodness and love for them. The enemy also knows man's fickleness. He knows the farther you are from your victories, the easier it is to forget the wilderness you came from and the miracles throughout the journey.

Memorials in Scripture come in many forms: feasts, altars, writings, and Scripture itself. Communion is also a memorial, a way to remember the sacrifice Jesus made for us. Your journals serve as a memorial of your wilderness journey with the Lord. **Your testimony is another memorial—your gift back to the Lord.**

Which brings us to your last assignment. You will build a memorial, a story of remembrance for everything the Lord has done in your life. This will not be an altar of brick and stone, but one forged from the sweat and tears of your journey.

And he took bread, and when he had given thanks, he broke it and gave it to them, saying, "This is my body, which is given for you. <u>Do this in remembrance of me</u>."
(Luke 22:19)

Truly, I say to you, wherever this gospel is proclaimed in the whole world, what she has done will also be told <u>in memory of her</u>. (Matthew 26:13)

Then the Lord said to Moses, "<u>Write this as a memorial in a book</u> and recite it in the ears of Joshua, that I will utterly blot out the memory of Amalek from under heaven." <u>And Moses built an altar and called the name of it, The Lord Is My Banner.</u>
(Exodus 17:14 – 15)

That this be a sign among you, so that when your children ask later, saying, "What do these stones mean to you?", then you shall say to them, "Because the waters of the Jordan were cut off before the ark of the covenant of the Lord; when it crossed the Jordan, the waters of the Jordan were cut off." So <u>these stones shall become a memorial to the sons of Israel forever</u>. (Joshua 4:4 – 7)

So these days were to be remembered and celebrated throughout every generation, every family, every province and every city; and these days of Purim were not to fail from among the Jews, <u>or their memory fade</u> from their descendants. (Esther 9:28)

Now this <u>day will be a memorial to you</u>, and you shall celebrate it as a feast to the Lord; throughout your generations you are to celebrate it as a permanent ordinance.
(Exodus 12:14)

Turn Your History into His Story

Rewrite your life story from the truth that the Lord has revealed to you. Your story will become a place to draw strength and truth. When you slip into old thinking, your story will serve to remind you of the Lord's transformative work. For others, it will become a testimony of encouragement, and a witness to the unbeliever. Use the guidelines that follow to rewrite your story and then share it with your coach.

- Gather your journals from your *Rebuilt* journey. Reread them. What you read will amaze you; it is worth the effort!

- Use your lists from your inventory to create a timeline of major events in your life.

- Write out the story of what happened during each life event.

- For each life event, write the truth as you now understand it.
  - Where was God in the event?
  - How did God use this event to benefit you or others?

- Mention how you felt then and describe your feelings now that you understand the truth!

Go!

Jesus gave us a great commission to make disciples. We are all expected by God to minister in the lives of others. He equips us with gifts and talents to help His Kingdom grow, but *Rebuilders* have something many do not have: a powerful testimony! Your coach can help you shorten your story to make a great testimony or pull from parts of your story to minister to someone's specific need. Even if your calling is not with *Rebuilt*, your testimony will be a powerful witness wherever the Lord leads you.

Serving with *Rebuilt*

If everyone who completes *Rebuilt* will coach only one person, the impact would be exponential. Your journey has equipped you to serve others and witness their lives transform as well. You continue growing even more when walking with another on their journey.

- We ask everyone who has completed their *Rebuilt* journey to write and share a video testimony to encourage others on their journey. You may choose how and where you share your testimony.

- Consider becoming a *Rebuilt* coach. We have training and materials available if you would like to lead others on a journey. The amazing thing about leading others is that you continue to grow right along with them!

- Consider becoming an online coach, guiding those who take the journey online.

- Consider joining the leadership team with *Rebuilt*. (You must first become a coach.)

Questions to Ponder

52.23) Rewrite your story and share it with your coach.

52.24) Do you have questions or concerns about sharing your testimony?

52.25) Do you see yourself serving with *Rebuilt*? How?

52.26) Write any questions you have for your coach about continuing forward.

Ask your coach for information about opportunities to serve with *Rebuilt!*

Appendix

Contents

How to Have Confidence

How can you be confident moving forward? The answer is not dependent on who you are, specific to a denomination, based on your gifts, your talents, or your success rate. Your confidence is based on and in the Lord, who has all knowledge and power. He gives gifts and talent to everyone,

You can find confidence in the power and purpose behind your abilities. The power comes from the Lord, and the purpose is His will. Those whose confidence lies in their talents or gifts are missing the One who enables the gifting. This is a counterfeit confidence.

The question is never "Are you able?" Rather it is "Do you have confidence in the God who makes you able?" When you have the master instructing you, is there anything you cannot do?

Picture a woman who fumbles around the kitchen, barely able to fix a simple meal. Her daughter is having a large graduation party and wants her to cook an enormous dinner for everyone. Yet the woman has never cooked such an elaborate meal.

Terrified, she realizes she does not have the money to hire a caterer for the party. But she knows a master chef, and she calls him for advice. He tells her everything she needs to buy, how to prepare the food, which seasonings to add, and how to cook it.

Now the woman has every confidence in her ability to fix the dinner. However, her confidence is not in her own talent but in the ability of the master chef guiding her.

To lack confidence in yourself is to lack confidence in God, the one guiding you through life. He is the master of everything, and there is nothing He cannot lead you through!

Battling Pride

I love photography! It is my favorite hobby, and one I wanted to make a career. Before shooting an event, I met with the client and asked questions until I had a detailed understanding of the final product they desired.

I knew precisely what they wanted before setting the stage for the shoot. Then, I began preparing the setting, creating the mood, and choosing the poses that would make my clients' photos into treasured and irreplaceable memories. My talent was often praised as I found beauty in the ordinary and captured those spontaneous moments that would otherwise be forever lost.

Why did I abandon my aspiration to be a professional photographer? Because it is exhausting! My clients constantly argued with me, pompously touting their flawed theories of how the stage should be set, what would work, and what I should do. They grumbled and complained, thinking they knew better how to produce the desired results.

But I was the photographer. I had the knowledge and experience. I knew the lighting, angles, and poses. I knew what they should wear and how they should stand. I understood the subtleties that make a photo great. After all, that was the reason they hired me.

This fictional scenario illustrates a truth in our relationship with God. He knows the beginning and the end and all that falls between. He knows how everything works because He created it all. Is there anything He can't do? Yet we argue and complain, thinking that His way will not provide the desired results. We think we know better than the professional and want it done our way. The Lord set the stage and put every piece in place. It is our job to swallow our pride and get out of His way.

Choose Your Diet

The problem with most diets is the nature of the diet. A diet designed for rapid transformation causes radical changes to the way you eat and live. But these changes are not sustainable. You cannot physically or mentally continue eating the same way. Eventually you will lose progress, regressing into old habits.

The perfect diet is one that alters your lifestyle. It doesn't leave you hungry or deprived. It is based on sustainability and balance. A good diet alters the way you eat forever. The changes are not as rapid, but you will find them permanent.

Jesus said to them, "I am the bread of life; whoever comes to me shall not hunger, and whoever believes in me shall never thirst. (John 6:35)

Consider your transformation with God like the perfect diet. You are eating the bread of life and drinking water that never leaves you thirsty. You experience breakthroughs that must be tested and tried so they become a solid, sustainable, change in you. Balance takes time. Remember, the urge you feel to rush back to the world's junk food is a test to strengthen you and bring your transformation to completion.

More than that, we rejoice in our sufferings, knowing that suffering produces endurance, and endurance produces character, and character produces hope. (Romans 5:3-4)

Don't try to run ahead of God! Expecting your first victory to be the end all, is like eating a fad diet. Seeking instant gratification leads to a superficial walk with Jesus. When it seems like you are being tested again and again, do not fall into frustration, condemnation, or shame. Have joy! God is molding you into His likeness. Embrace the process. Stop fighting Him! You can't change yourself, but God can. And your acceptance and cooperation make the process much easier.

*The authentic work of God is not instant gratification,
rather it is sustainable and eternal.*

Want the Real Thing!

Passing the Test

Scripture says that we are tested through our trials and tribulations. What does this mean? Why would God test us, and how do we know if we pass or fail a test? We find the answer in the book of Job.

And if they are bound in chains and caught in the cords of affliction, then he declares to them their work and their transgressions, that they are behaving arrogantly. He opens their ears to instruction and commands that they return from iniquity... He delivers the afflicted by their affliction and opens their ear by adversity. He also allured you out of distress into a broad place where there was no cramping, and what was set on your table was full of fatness. (Job 8 – 10, 15 – 16)

In this passage, Elihu explains how the Lord uses our trials. Job experienced some of the hardest trials depicted in Scripture. He did not understand why, as a righteous man, he was suffering so much pain and loss. His wife told him to curse God and die, and his friends tried to convince him that his suffering was due to some sin, so he should simply repent. Instead of defending the Lord's righteousness in the situation, Job began to defend his righteousness to the people accusing him of wrongdoing. Despite his grief and pain, he was concerned with the opinions of man, and thus he became lifted in pride. Then Elihu comes forth and speaks truth to Job, leading him to repentance and restoration.

From Elihu's message to Job, we can see that God uses the trials, temptations, and tribulations we face to get our attention. When we are prepared to listen, He shows us the iniquity in our hearts. The Lord speaks through the chains of our affliction and opens our ears to hear his words through adversity. Then, when we have learned from the test, the Lord can restore and bless us.

That which seems like failure, is a growing process. The only way to fail is if the test does not result in understanding and growth. We will continue to be tested through adversity until we are perfected in our character.

For you know that the testing of your faith produces steadfastness. And let steadfastness have its full effect, that you may be perfect and complete, lacking in nothing. (James 1:3 – 4)

Fear vs Truth

He who has an ear, let him hear! Do you ever feel defeated, condemned? Do you ever ask yourself, "What is wrong with me?", "Why am I going through this again?", or "Why do I keep failing?". Do you still feel like God's word is truth for other people, but not for you? Or, perhaps, you feel like God is not the problem, but you are. You just are too messed up or too bad for God to fix.

If you have any of these thoughts, you likely have shame. Remember, guilt is when you have done something bad, but shame is when you believe you are bad. We all have a sin nature that makes us wicked. The truth is that Jesus died to overcome our sin. We do not own that identity.

God calls you righteous through your faith, your repentance, and the blood of Jesus. He has given you a purpose, a future, and a hope. **But how can He use someone for His kingdom, who feels like they are unqualified to be used?**

FEAR	TRUTH
F – *False*	T – *True*
E – *Evidence*	R – *Reality*
A – *Appearing*	U – *Unfolding*
R – *Real*	T – *Through*
	H – *Him*

You must come out of agreement with the lies. You can choose to believe what God says is good and evil or choose to believe your own ideas of good and evil. **Who are you to say you are bad when God says you are righteous?**

It is the Holy Spirit's job to convict you of sin. *The enemy's tactic is to cause you to doubt and question "What if I can't see what's wrong with me or if I am wrong?"* **Don't seek the wrong, seek the Lord.** *He will bring your sin to your attention. Once he shows you, it is your job to repent from it and allow Him to correct it. God is faithful to finish what He started in you! Ask God if there is any way in you that displeases Him and trust Him to reveal it to you. It is not your job to discover what the Spirit has not revealed.*

The Choice of Two

<u>See, I have set before you today life and goodness, as well as death and disaster.</u>
For I am commanding you today to love the LORD your God, to walk in His ways, and to keep His commandments, statutes, and ordinances, so that you may live and increase, and the LORD your God may bless you in the land that you are entering to possess. But if your heart turns away and you do not listen, but are drawn away to bow down to other gods and worship them, I declare to you today that you will surely perish; you shall not prolong your days in the land that you are crossing the Jordan to possess. I call heaven and earth as witnesses against you today that **<u>I have set before you life and death, blessing and cursing. Therefore choose life,</u>** *so that you and your descendants may live. (Deuteronomy 30:15-19 BSB)*

God does not change.

For I the Lord do not change... (Malachi 3:6)

Jesus Christ is the same yesterday and today and forever. (Hebrews 13:8)

The counsel of the Lord stands forever, the plans of his heart to all generations. (Psalm 33:11)

Choose life and live or choose death and cursing. This is the same choice presented to the first man and woman. The choice represented by two trees in the center of the garden. Choose the first, the Tree of Life, from which eternal life flowed, or choose the Tree of the Knowledge of Good and Evil, which led to death and separation from God. This is the choice He presented the Israelites as they entered the promised land. **God offers us the same choice today,** that He has given humanity since the beginning of our existence.

In the garden, mankind had dominion over everything, yet **there was one thing that God never allowed mankind to do – to decide for themselves what was good and evil.** He was the author of good, and He alone defined it.

The way the story is told in children's storybooks may make you think that this tree had some magical power to instantly reveal knowledge of good and evil by eating its fruit, but that is not exactly what happened.

<u>When the woman saw that the tree was good</u> for food and <u>pleasing to the eyes,</u> and that <u>it was desirable</u> for obtaining wisdom, she took the fruit and ate it. She also gave some to her husband who was with her, and he ate it. (Genesis 3:6-7)

At that moment, doubting God's truth, the woman decided she knew the tree was good. She decided that what she thought was good and desirable was better than what God thought was good and desirable, and it led to a curse and the death of her sinless nature. Her choice was pride, lack of faith, lack of trust, leaning on her own understanding, and blatant sin – disobedience to God. These are the same things we struggle with today.

Each moment of each day we are presented with the choice to choose life and live.

Everything we deal with in this life can be boiled down to the same choice. Do we choose our own idols and desires, that which we want and think is good, or do we choose what God says is good and trust His thoughts and understanding regarding what is right?

Galatians 5 shows us the contrast between acts that come from God's way of thinking and our sin nature's way of thinking. If we think in our flesh (sin nature) we choose death. If we choose the mind of Christ, we choose life!

The acts of the flesh are obvious: sexual immorality, impurity, and debauchery; idolatry and sorcery; hatred, discord, jealousy, and rage; rivalries, divisions, factions, and envy; drunkenness, orgies, and the like. I warn you, as I did before, that those who practice such things will not inherit the kingdom of God. But the fruit of the Spirit is love, joy, peace, patience, kindness, goodness, faithfulness, gentleness, and self-control.
Against such things there is no law. (Galatians 5:19-22)

Sorcery is attempting to make what you want to happen in your power (or Satan's power). Hatred is something you don't want or like. Discord is creating problems to get your way. Jealousy is the fear of losing what is yours to another. Rage and anger burn in your heart when you become offended. **All of these things allow your own desires and understanding to define what is good, instead of believing what God says is good**.

We are not much different than the serpent, quick to twist God's truth to fit our circumstances and desires. Therefore we must take off the ways of our old life and old ways of thinking and put on the mind of Christ. We must not lean on our understanding, but acknowledge God in all our ways, and take every thought and feeling captive and make it obedient to Christ.

God alone had the right to determine good and evil. He alone is just, and His justice is right. When we do not agree with His actions – **HE IS RIGHT.** When we decide for ourselves how things should or should not be, or what is or is not good **we are trying to take the place of God and usurp His authority.**

When we value something as more important (better) than God or His ways we choose death. When we set aside our own desires and wisdom to follow God, His commandments, and His ways, we choose life. Not sure which choice you are making? Examine your fruit! What do you do when you don't get what you want, or when things don't go how you think they should go? What do you do when you are frustrated because things are hard and you are impatient?

Choose to believe God is good and trust in the goodness of His ways.
It's just that simple!

The Root of All Emotion

We have an enemy that loves to play on the emotions of our sin nature, and a God who is trying to transform our sin nature into one that looks like Him. We are caught in a war of thoughts, a battle between God and Satan fighting for our soul.

Think of it as if you are the object of a huge custody battle with two parents each demanding full right to you, each claiming you belong to them. Every day, the devil stands before the court making accusations, testifying of all the ways you mess up and all the reasons you belong to him. He has gone to great lengths to tempt you to reject God and His ways. **Satan is fear** and **lies**.

On the other side of the court, Jesus stands with the custody documents. He owns you and your debt has been paid in full. The cost, His life. He counters every argument of the enemy with your righteousness, all your wrongs justified for a price. **God is love**, a parent who is just and deals only in **truth**.

Our emotions send us messages that catch us up in a war of thoughts between these two opposites. Messages that bounce between truth and lies, depending on their source, distorting God's truth with a twisted understanding that leaves us double minded. It is hard to see truth clearly when our emotions seem to confirm the enemy's convincing lies.

Of course, it's complicated... Or is it?

In psychology, there is a claim that **every emotion we feel, is rooted in one of two sources, either love or fear**. This aligns with scripture. Emotions speak messages to your mind. An emotion rooted in love comes from the Lord and is truth, and an emotion rooted in fear comes from the enemy and is a lie. It may seem simple to identify from which source an emotion flows, but **many times it is not.** Therefore, we must take emotions captive, examine them, and submit them to the word of God, and never rely on them to guide our thoughts and actions.

Anger is an emotion that you may quickly identify as being rooted in fear, but God says in scripture to love what he loves and hate what he hates, and God himself gets angry. Scripture says not to be angry because the anger of man is not righteous, and also to be angry – but not sin in your anger. This is because Anger **can come from either source**.

How do you win the battle of your emotions? Be perfected in Love!

So we have come to know and to believe the love that God has for us. God is love, and whoever abides in love abides in God, and God abides in him. By this is love perfected with us, so that we may have confidence for the day of judgment, because as he is so also are we in this world. There is no fear in love, but perfect love casts out fear. For fear has to do with punishment, and whoever fears has not been perfected in love. We love because he first loved us. (1 John 4:16-19)

Three ways to find the source of your emotion

1. **To find the source ask yourself why?**
   If the reason for your emotion lines up with God's thoughts and ways, it is likely based in love. If not, it may be based in fear.
   Here are a couple of examples.

   - **Why am I angry?**
     Are you angry at unrighteousness, or was there a true injustice? Were God or His ways being disrespected? This anger may be rooted in love.
     Did something not go your way? Did you dislike an outcome or result? Did someone make you feel bad or insecure? This is anger probably based in fear.

   - **Why do I love?**
     Is my love for a person sacrificial? Is it patient and slow to anger, kind and not self-seeking? Do I love because I want to grow with another in God, give myself, invest my time, and share my life and resources with them? This love is based out of God's love.
     Do I love them because they have a lot in common with me and they fill a missing spot in my life? Because I don't want to be lonely, or they fill a lack in my life? Am I looking for something specific from them like protection or security? Do they fill a need? This love may be based out of fear.

   - **Why do I feel proud?**
     Is my confidence because I know God makes me able, or in the quality of person God is transforming in me? If your confidence is in the Lord, it is based in Love.
     God warns against pride. Do you feel a need to boast or put others down to make yourself appear better? Do you feel insecure? Do you fear failing? Do you think you are entitled? Do you need to prove yourself? Are you trying to be good enough? Do you think others are not as good as you? This is fear-based pride.

2. **To find the source examine the message you hear in your mind.**
   Do the messages you hear make you feel loved, love others, feel compassion, have joy, give you confidence or purpose? These are messages from love.
   Do the messages make you feel defeated, hopeless, fearful, or condemned? Are they selfish thoughts or do they appeal to your flesh? Do you feel like a failure, or fear the opinions of man? These are messages based in fear.

3. **To find the source examine your fruit, the actions, that result from your thoughts and emotions.**
   Do your actions bring glory to the Lord? Do they build others up and biblically cover their sin? Do they follow God's commandments? They are love-based.
   Do they cause others harm or tear people down? Do they puff you up with pride? Do they indulge your flesh? These are based in fear.

I Shall Not Want

Why did God's people in the Old Testament continually turn to false gods, even though the Lord was faithful to them? He gave them astounding victories over their enemies, blessings, and riches. In the wilderness, their clothes did not wear out and provision fell from the sky. Yet, they were never satisfied, always wanting, serving other gods and idols trying to satisfy the desires of their flesh. This angered God.

> **Because you did not serve the LORD your God <u>with joyfulness and gladness of heart</u>, because of the abundance of all things, you shall serve your enemies in hunger and thirst, in nakedness, and lacking everything. And he will put a yoke of iron on your neck until he has destroyed you. (Deuteronomy 28:47-48)**

When the people of Israel wanted a king like the world, God's heart wanted David to be king of Israel. David became Israel's second king. It was a difficult journey to the throne, yet God knew that David would act according to His will.

> **And when he had removed him [Saul], he raised up David to be their king, of whom he testified and said, 'I have found in David the son of Jesse a man after my heart, who will do all my will.' (Acts 13:22)**

David made some serious mistakes during his time as king. He encountered some terrifying and heartbreaking situations and cried out to the Lord, but he never grumbled against the Lord. He always acknowledged God's goodness and justice. He never accused God of being unfair or complained about His instruction. He always deferred his situations, his sin, his feelings, and his fear to the Lord's just judgment. He trusted God completely.

David stayed humble. He showed mercy and love to his enemies. He loved the Lord with every bit of his heart and worshipped Him with all he had in him. David was never afraid of the outcome. He was willing to lay down his crown and step away from the throne, knowing if it was God's will, He would bring him back.

> **For David had done what was right in the eyes of the LORD and had not turned aside from anything the LORD commanded all the days of his life, except in the matter of Uriah the Hittite. (1 Kings 15:5 BSB)**

In the 23rd Psalm, David writes, "The Lord is my shepherd, **<u>I shall not want</u>**". He trusted God to provide, but also treated this as a command. He shall not – will not – want. He **shall not want more** than God gives Him. He **shall not want his own will** to be done. He **shall not want his way**. He **shall be satisfied** with what the Lord has given. Having the Lord with him was enough for him. He feared the Lord and knew He was sovereign. He accepted that God gives and takes away, and He is right and just for doing so.

David knew not to complain or question God's decisions, even when it was unpleasant for him. He also knew He could take his complaints before the Lord, but that He must do it humbly, knowing that God's will was perfect.

Do all things without grumbling or questioning, that you may be blameless and innocent, children of God without blemish in the midst of a crooked and twisted generation, among whom you shine as lights in the world, Philippians 2:14-15

David knew Israel's tendencies to run away from God to serve idols. As king, he would not let that happen, but Israel was not much different than we are today. When they couldn't get what they wanted from God's ways, they tried to get it elsewhere.

"So many today are not content with our perfect God. They think they can tweak Him and His commands to fit their mold, their agenda, and their ways. From the outside many appear to be living the so-called Christian life, but something is not quite right. It doesn't quite click because instead of leading others away from sin, there tends to be a leading towards sin, whether in idolatry or other sin.

There must be an opening of our eyes to see all that the Lord has given us, <u>to be content</u>, to obey His commands, and to see the Lord correctly that His ways are perfect and true, as well as see ourselves rightly.

Throughout the Old Testament I have noticed God repeating 'Follow my commands and statutes and walk in my ways'; it's a command He gives. There is no veering to the right or the left and doing it slightly our way, why? Because our way leads to death; His way leads to life! It saddens me to see so many deceived, as the saying goes, 'We can have our cake and eat it too' type Christians out there."

–Alysha Allen (Used with permission)

Our God is a god of wrath against the wicked, but He is also the God of grace that made a way, and guides us along that way, to his righteousness. He is the God who has done for us what we could not do for ourselves – save us from our wicked nature. Yes, this is the God who gave you your life at the cost of His own son's life. The God who provides all your needs, protects you, and comforts you in your trials. Why wouldn't He be offended by your complaints?

It was also about these that Enoch, the seventh from Adam, prophesied, saying, "Behold, the Lord comes with ten thousands of his holy ones, to execute judgment on all and to convict all the ungodly of all their deeds of ungodliness that they have committed in such an ungodly way, and of all the harsh things that ungodly sinners have spoken against him." <u>These are grumblers, malcontents, following their own sinful desires; they are loud-mouthed boasters, showing favoritism to gain advantage.</u> (Jude 1:14-16)

God wants cheerful givers, with hearts of gratitude. He abhors grumbling. When we complain about our lives, our situations, others, or ourselves, we are complaining against God.

And Moses said, "When the Lord gives you in the evening meat to eat and in the morning bread to the full, because the Lord has heard your grumbling that you grumble against him—what are we? Your grumbling is not against us but against the Lord." (Exodus 16:8)

When you declared that God was Lord (or master) of your life, you gave up your right to be lord. When you told Him, "You will be my God!", that means that you can no longer be your own god. What right do you have to complain when your life belongs to Him?

- ***For the sake of Christ, then, I am content with weaknesses, insults, hardships, persecutions, and calamities. For when I am weak, then I am strong. (2 Corinthians 12:10)***

- ***Not that I am speaking of being in need, for I have learned in whatever situation I am to be content. I know how to be brought low, and I know how to abound. In any and every circumstance, I have learned the secret of facing plenty and hunger, abundance and need. (Philippians 4:11-12)***

- ***Keep your life free from love of money, and be content with what you have, for he has said, "I will never leave you nor forsake you." (Hebrews 13:5)***

- ***Now there is great gain in godliness with contentment, for we brought nothing into the world, and we cannot take anything out of the world. But if we have food and clothing, with these we will be content. (1 Timothy 6:6-8)***

- ***And he said to them, "Take care, and be on your guard against all covetousness, for one's life does not consist in the abundance of his possessions." (Luke 12:15)***

- ***Now there is great gain in godliness with contentment. (1 Timothy 6:6)***

- ***"Blessed are those who hunger and thirst for righteousness, for they shall be satisfied. (Matthew 5:6)***

- ***The fear of the Lord leads to life, and whoever has it rests satisfied; he will not be visited by harm. (Proverbs 19:23)***

- ***Better is a handful of quietness than two hands full of toil and a striving after wind. (Ecclesiastes 4:6)***

I Shall Not Want

Fear of God and Man

To Fear, or Not to Fear?

The Lord commands at least 82 times in scripture that we should "fear the Lord" or have a "fear of the Lord". It is in the purpose behind the first commandment he gives to the people in Deuteronomy. In Isaiah 11, the fear of the Lord is one of the Spirits of God.

That you may <u>fear the Lord your God</u>, you and your son and your son's son, by keeping all his statutes and his commandments, which I command you, all the days of your life, and that your days may be long…. You shall love the Lord your God with all your heart and with all your soul and with all your might. And these words that I command you today shall be on your heart." (Deuteronomy 6:2, 5-6)

There shall come forth a shoot from the stump of Jesse, and a branch from his roots shall bear fruit. And the Spirit of the Lord shall rest upon him, the Spirit of wisdom and understanding, the Spirit of counsel and might, the Spirit of knowledge <u>and the fear of the Lord</u>. And his delight shall be in the fear of the Lord. He shall not judge by what his eyes see, or decide disputes by what his ears hear. (Isaiah 11:1-3)

So, does God really want us to be terrified of him? Scripture often tells us not to be afraid. This can be confusing for believers. What exactly is the fear of the Lord?

To those in the world, the fear of the Lord should be terrifying.

And the fear of the Lord fell upon all the kingdoms of the lands that were around Judah, and they made no war against Jehoshaphat. (2 Chronicles 17:10)

For us, however, it is knowing the **fear of not being in right standing with the Lord**. It is **knowing the might and power and righteousness of our God**. It is **standing in awe** of who He is and what He does. It is **knowing He gives and takes away**; He is **a just and righteous judge**. It is **accepting His discipline** and **hating sin**. It is **trusting the Lord's sovereignty** in every situation in our lives. It is **believing** His word is true, and that He will do what He says He will do. **It is humility**, keeping God in His rightful place as God, and us in our rightful place as His servants. **Knowing we are the clay – not the Potter**. It is **loving Him more than self**, putting **Him first** in our lives. It is **obedience** and **wisdom**.

"See now that I, even I, am he, and there is no god beside me; I kill and I make alive; I wound and I heal; and there is none that can deliver out of my hand." (Deuteronomy 30:39)

You will say to me then, "Why does he still find fault? For who can resist his will?" But who are you, O man, to answer back to God? Will what is molded say to its molder, "Why have you made me like this?" Has the potter no right over the clay, to make out of the same lump one vessel for honorable use and another for dishonorable use? What if God, desiring to show his wrath and to make known his power, has endured with much patience vessels of wrath prepared for destruction, in order to make known the riches of his glory for vessels of mercy, which he has prepared beforehand for glory. (Romans 9:19- 23)

Why do you serve the Lord? Do you serve from an obligation? Do you serve to avoid hell? Or do you serve Him because you fear him and love him and know He alone is worthy of your love?

"Hear, O Israel: The Lord our God, the Lord is one. You shall love the Lord your God with all your heart and with all your soul and with all your might. And these words that I command you today shall be on your heart. You shall teach them diligently to your children, and shall talk of them when you sit in your house, and when you walk by the way, and when you lie down, and when you rise. (Deuteronomy 6:4-7)

Fear the Lord – Not Man

Why fear the opinions of people? Why are you worried about impressing your coworkers, boss, neighbors, or friends? Do you fear their rejection if your thoughts, words, or actions offend them? They have no power over your soul. **Trying to please others often puts you at odds with God.** *It is better to fear the Lord and His thoughts about you than any man's opinions. It is better to worry about offending God than offending people. Better to risk the rejection of man than rejection from the Lord!*

And do not fear those who kill the body but cannot kill the soul. Rather fear him who can destroy both soul and body in hell. (Matthew 10:28)

I tell you, my friends, do not fear those who kill the body, and after that have nothing more that they can do. But I will warn you whom to fear: fear him who, after he has killed, has authority to cast into hell. Yes, I tell you, fear him! (Luke 12:4-5)

For am I now seeking the approval of man, or of God? Or am I trying to please man? If I were still trying to please man, I would not be a servant of Christ. (Galatians 1:10)

The fear of man lays a snare, but whoever trusts in the Lord is safe. (Proverbs 29:25)

Saul said to Samuel, "I have sinned, for I have transgressed the commandment of the Lord and your words, because I feared the people and obeyed their voice. (1 Samuel 15:24)

So we can confidently say, "The Lord is my helper; I will not fear; what can man do to me?" (Hebrews 13:6)

The Lord is on my side; I will not fear. What can man do to me? (Psalm 118:6)

When I am afraid, I put my trust in you. In God, whose word I praise, in God I trust; I shall not be afraid. What can flesh do to me? (Psalm 56:3-4)

But even if you should suffer for righteousness' sake, you will be blessed. Have no fear of them, nor be troubled. (1 Peter 3:14)

"I, I am he who comforts you; who are you that you are afraid of man who dies, of the son of man who is made like grass". (Isaiah 51:12)

The Fear of the Lord Defined

The Fear of the Lord is:

- *A requirement – **(Deuteronomy 10:12)***
  And now, Israel, what does the Lord your God require of you, but to fear the Lord your God, to walk in all his ways, to love him, to serve the Lord your God with all your heart and with all your soul.

- *Hatred of evil – **(Proverbs 8:13)***
  The fear of the Lord is hatred of evil. Pride and arrogance and the way of evil and perverted speech I hate.

- *Respecting God's authority (obedience) – **(Genesis 22:12)***
  He said, "Do not lay your hand on the boy or do anything to him, for now I know that you fear God, seeing you have not withheld your son, your only son, from me."

- *Wisdom – **(Psalm 111:10)***
  The fear of the Lord is the beginning of wisdom; all those who practice it have a good understanding. His praise endures forever!

- *Awe – **(Psalm 33:8)***
  Let all the earth fear the Lord; let all the inhabitants of the world stand in awe of him!

- *Reverent fear – **(Hebrews 11:7)***
  By faith Noah, being warned by God concerning events as yet unseen, in reverent fear constructed an ark for the saving of his household. By this he condemned the world and became an heir of the righteousness that comes by faith.

- *Terror on His enemies – **(2 Chronicles 17:10)***
  And the fear of the Lord fell upon all the kingdoms of the lands that were around Judah, and they made no war against Jehoshaphat.

- *Fountain of Life – **(Proverbs 14:27)***
  The fear of the Lord is a fountain of life, that one may turn away from the snares of death.

- *Strong Confidence – **(Proverbs 14:26)***
  In the fear of the Lord one has strong confidence, and his children will have a refuge.

- *Complete Holiness – **(2 Corinthians 7:1)***
  Since we have these promises, beloved, let us cleanse ourselves from every defilement of body and spirit, bringing holiness to completion in the fear of God.

- *Trust – **(Psalm 115:11)***
  You who fear the Lord, trust in the Lord! He is their help and their shield.

- *Rewarded with Blessings, Friendship of the Lord, No lack, and God's compassion.*
  (Psalm 112:1) Blessed is the man who fears the Lord, who greatly delights in his commandments!
  (Psalm 25:14) The friendship of the Lord is for those who fear him
  (Psalm 34:9) Those who fear him have no lack!
  (Psalm 103:13) The Lord shows compassion to those who fear him.
  (Proverbs 22:4) The reward for humility and fear of the Lord is riches and honor and life.

The Self-god

For rebellion is as the sin of witchcraft, and stubbornness is as iniquity and idolatry.
(1 Samuel 15:23 BSB)

As a Christian, you probably believe you are far from the sin of idolatry and witchcraft. Yet, if you are like most people, you have stubborn and rebellious moments. The verse above may have you wondering, "What exactly is idolatry and witchcraft?"

Witchcraft involves a manipulation of circumstances powered by the demonic. It is often blatant occultic practices – most likely things you don't do. Yet, **at the heart** of witchcraft is the desire to know the future and control events that are not ours to control, abilities that belong only to the Lord. It is the desire to be in control that causes rebellion. Can you see the similarity to witchcraft? The Lord looks at the heart. **A rebellious heart is the same condition of the heart willing to perform witchcraft.**

In rebellion, we attempt to make situations line up with our desires instead of seeking the Lord's will. We attempt to control how our life will go, instead of accepting the Lord's will for our life. We try to manipulate circumstances to our benefit and our ways, instead of relying on God's ways. We want to fast-track the path we are on or define our destiny as we want it. We may even attempt to control or manipulate another person's will to line up with our will. This is the core purpose of witchcraft.

Do you grumble and complain? How are you unsatisfied with life? What do you try to control? The answers to these questions can help you spot rebellion in your heart.

Idolatry is not the same as witchcraft. I searched scripture to define idolatry and found Colossians 3:5, but I noticed some differences within the translations.

Colossians 3:5

Therefore put to death your members which are on the earth: fornication, uncleanness, passion, evil desire, and covetousness, which is idolatry. (New King James Version)

Put to death therefore what is earthly in you: sexual immorality, impurity, passion, evil desire, and covetousness, which is idolatry. (English Standard Version)

You must put to death, then, the earthly desires at work in you, such as sexual immorality, indecency, lust, evil passions, and greed (for greed is a form of idolatry). (Good News Translation)

So put to death the sinful, earthly things lurking within you. Have nothing to do with sexual immorality, impurity, lust, and evil desires. Don't be greedy, for a greedy person is an idolater, worshiping the things of this world. (New Living Translation)

The first two translations appear to give a list of things that are idolatry, but the last two state it is only greed. **To find out if all these works of the flesh were idolatry or if it was just greed, I looked up how the phrase "which is idolatry" was translated from the Greek.**

The word used for "which" was hétis (hay-tis); it can mean whoever, anyone, or someone of such a nature, but this particular usage of the word serves to give a reason. It is equivalent to saying, "seeing that he did this" or "inasmuch as he did that".

The word used for "idolatry" is eidólolatria (i-do-lol-at-ri'-ah). This is fairly straight forward. The definition is image worship; the service (worship) of an image (an idol).

So, Colossians 3:5 could be read to say:

> *Put to death therefore what is earthly in you: sexual immorality, impurity, passion, evil desire, and covetousness, **seeing that you are worshipping an image***

It could also just as accurately be translated:

> *Put to death therefore what is earthly in you: sexual immorality, impurity, passion, evil desire, and covetousness, **inasmuch as you are in the service of an idol.***

Let's read 1 Samuel 15:23 again.

"For rebellion is as the sin of witchcraft, and stubbornness is as iniquity and idolatry."

Witchcraft is a response to idolatry just as rebellion is an action that results from stubbornness. *God is sovereign. He is in control, but we want control. We want to change situations to benefit our will. We want our will to be done on earth. Our stubbornness is equated to idolatry. It is the heart condition that promotes the rebellion. Our acts of rebellion are like performing witchcraft. Being stubborn against the ways of God is the worship of a false god or idol.* ***So, rebellion is an <u>act of worship</u> to a false god, and the god is you.*** *When you seek knowledge, power, or spirituality apart from God, it is idolatry, and puts you in rebellion to God's sovereignty.*

Satan is full of pride and hate. He hates you because you have a resemblance of God. If he can divert your heart away from worshipping the true God and entice you with the idea of self-power, control, self-realization, or spiritual enlightenment apart from submission to the authority of the Lord Almighty, He destroys the image of God in you eternally.

The Anti-God Battle

Satan excels in counterfeiting what God does. Do you remember the magicians, who by demonic power, created counterfeits of the miracles Moses performed before Pharaoh? Today, he continues to counterfeit the authentic.

Mankind was created in a divine nature, not as gods, but without sin, like God. In the Garden of Eden, mankind walked with God, and He gave mankind all authority and dominion of the earth, except one thing. He told Adam the one thing he may not do was to eat of the tree of the knowledge of good and evil. The one thing God said mankind could not do was to decide for himself what was good or evil. Once we decided for ourselves what was good and bad, we also decided what was right and wrong, thus creating our own morality apart from the Lord.

We continue in this same sin today. We decide for ourselves what is right and wrong, and we become the arbiters of justice. We redefine what God calls good and corrupt it – we create a counterfeit, in the same way Satan creates counterfeits.

Satan wanted to rule; he wanted God's throne. He wanted to show himself mightier than God. **In the garden, Satan created the beginning of an army of servants who would go fourth counterfeiting God's good design and corrupting His plan, His will, and His word for generations.**

So, now we see why the Lord is right and just to destroy the wicked. Why He is right to demand no other God before Him, and that He is sovereign. His jealousy is righteous. His ways are good because even before he created the opportunity to choose wrong, he made the escape route. He had the plan of salvation in place before the foundations of the world were laid.

> **For if these qualities are yours and are increasing, they keep you from being ineffective or unfruitful in the knowledge of our Lord Jesus Christ. <u>For whoever lacks these qualities is so nearsighted that he is blind, having forgotten that he was cleansed from his former sins.</u>**
> **(2 Peter 1-8-9)**

When you choose the ways of your flesh – or your own understanding, seeking knowledge or control outside of God – you become blind, near-sighted – only looking at the situation right in front of you, or dissecting the details of a situation into oblivion trying to make sense of or control something that is not yours to know or control. You forget who you are and who you belong to. God is your master, your lord. He owns you. He paid a hefty price, the life of His Son, for you. And He is Sovereign.

The Anti-Christ Flesh

If worshipping your flesh is idolatry and idolatry is the worship of an image, what image are you worshipping when you indulge your flesh? You might say your own image, you are worshiping self. We are made in the image of God – yet these things are contrary to God, or anti-God. Therefore, the image we are worshipping is an anti-god image.

> **For the mind that is set on the flesh is hostile to God,**
> **for it does not submit to God's law; indeed, it cannot. (Romans 8:7)**

> **For the desires of the flesh are against the Spirit, and the desires of the Spirit are against the flesh, for these are opposed to each other, to keep you from doing the things you want to do. (Galatians 5:17)**

Who owns you? You are either owned by your sin and the world, which falls under the dominion of the enemy, or you are owned by God. The world hates you. It is out for itself. Your sin deceives you. It cares only about the moment and cannot perceive what is truly good. The only power your sin has is to destroy and decay. It rots your soul and

266

kills you. God on the other hand, loves you. He plans a future for you, an eternal future. He gives you hope, peace and joy. He wants good for you and is generous and selfless.

Do you not know that if you present yourselves to anyone as obedient slaves, you are slaves of the one whom you obey, either of sin, which leads to death, or of obedience, which leads to righteousness? (Romans 6:16)

What are the things of the flesh that we worship?

"Now the works of the flesh are evident: sexual immorality, impurity, sensuality, idolatry, sorcery, enmity, strife, jealousy, fits of anger, rivalries, dissensions, divisions, envy, drunkenness, orgies, and things like these. I warn you, as I warned you before, that those who do such things will not inherit the kingdom of God." (Galatians 5:19-21)

If you are causing dissention and divisions, gossip, attention seeking, could it be that power and acceptance are your gods? Is sex your god? Rivalries and fits of anger? Could success and money be your gods? What about your phone? Social media? Entertainment? Your job or your status? Perhaps it is your friends or your family that are your god? Anything at all that you **put above** *God,* **value more** *than God**, take time away from God** to do, or that you would* **rebel against God** *to do, that is your idol.*

We are to love God with **all** *our heart, mind, and soul. When we are acting in our flesh, being disobedient to God, we are against him.* **If we are not for Him, we are against Him.** *We are not loving God; we are loving the world and become an enemy of God.* **We are not worshipping Christ. We are worshipping the anti-Christ.**

I am **not** *talking about worshipping the man called the Anti-christ who is coming to wreak havoc on this world. I am speaking about you. Every idol mentioned above glorifies you. The one being worshipped is your own self above God.*

Do not love the world or anything in the world. If anyone loves the world, the love of the Father is not in him. For all that is in the world—the desires of the flesh, the desires of the eyes, and the pride of life—is not from the Father but from the world. The world is passing away, along with its desires; but whoever does the will of God remains forever. Children, it is the last hour; and just as you have heard that the antichrist is coming, so now many antichrists have appeared. This is how we know it is the last hour. <u>They went out from us, but they did not belong to us. For if they had belonged to us, they would have remained with us.</u> But their departure made it clear that none of them belonged to us. (1 John 2 15-19)

This scripture speaks of people in the church being exposed and separated in the last hour, which we are certainly in. Many people will come with a form of godliness and an outward appearance of Christ, but inwardly deny the power of the true God and are ravenous wolves. People worshipping self and their flesh more than the Lord will be separated from the fold because their hearts are not genuinely for the Lord. They have not circumcised the flesh of their heart. **Is this you?**

The Self-lover

God Respects Himself

God knows He is worthy of respect, there is none equal to him, none who compares to Him. He sees Himself as worthy, and He demands the respect he deserves. God loves Himself, and commands us to love Him also, as well as ourselves and others. You cannot love your neighbor as yourself if you do not love yourself.

Love Your Neighbor <u>as Yourself</u>

"Loving others as yourself" shows us how we are to treat ourselves as much as it shows us how to treat others. You may know it is wrong to harm another person with your words, yet you harm yourself with your own thoughts and words. You may cover over another person's wrongs in love yet beat yourself up for your own wrongs. You may forgive another and not forgive yourself. Or vice-versa. You may ignore your faults and blame others. You may gossip about others to build your own confidence and cover your own flaws. Neither are love. Thus, loving others as yourself is a command to love both other people and you.

Don't take vengeance on or bear a grudge against any of your people; rather, love your neighbor as yourself; I am Adonai. (Leviticus 19:18)

Rather, treat the foreigner staying with you like the native-born among you — you are to love him as yourself, for you were foreigners in the land of Egypt; I am Adonai your God. (Leviticus 19:34)

'And you shall love the Lord your God with all your heart and with all your soul and with all your mind and with all your strength.' The second is this: 'You shall love your neighbor as yourself.' There is no other commandment greater than these. (Mark 12:30-31)

And he said to him, "You shall love the Lord your God with all your heart and with all your soul and with all your mind. This is the great and first commandment. And a second is like it: You shall love your neighbor as yourself. (Matthew 22:37-39)

Honor your father and mother, and, You shall love your neighbor as yourself. (Matthew 19:19)

And he answered, "You shall love the Lord your God with all your heart and with all your soul and with all your strength and with all your mind, and your neighbor as yourself." (Luke 10:27)

If you really fulfill the royal law according to the Scripture, "You shall love your neighbor as yourself," you are doing well. (James 2:8)

For the whole law is fulfilled in one word: "You shall love your neighbor as yourself." (Galatians 5:14)

For the commandments, "Don't commit adultery," "Don't murder," "Don't steal," "Don't covet," and any others are summed up in this one rule: "Love your neighbor as yourself." (Romans 13:9)

Loving Yourself vs Being a Lover of Self

There is a distinction between loving yourself and being lovers of self.

But understand this, that in the last days there will come times of difficulty. For people will be lovers of self, lovers of money, proud, arrogant, abusive, disobedient to their parents, ungrateful, unholy, heartless, unappeasable, slanderous, without self-control, brutal, not loving good, treacherous, reckless, swollen with conceit, lovers of pleasure rather than lovers of God, having the appearance of godliness, but denying its power. Avoid such people. (2 Timothy 3:1-5)

God condemns being a lover of self. The difference between loving yourself and being a lover of self is how you treat others and the value you place on your eternal soul.

Whoever gets sense loves his own soul; he who keeps understanding will discover good. (Proverbs 19:8)

What are you loving when you love your soul? You love the new creation you are becoming in Christ. You love your eternal soul, your eternal existence with God. You place eternity as having a higher value than this life. Understanding this you will "discover good". You will keep the Lord's commands because you love your soul enough to protect it from eternal consequences.

If you are loving yourself, you respect yourself and want others to treat you well. You, therefore, can treat other people the way you would like to be treated. When you love yourself, you are not in competition with others. You can give them honor, because you know that you are honorable and do not need the recognition. Therefore, you can show others a high regard, esteem them, build them up, without taking credit for yourself.

"So whatever you wish that others would do to you, do also to them, for this is the Law and the Prophets. (Matthew 7:12)

Do nothing from selfish ambition or conceit, but in humility count others more significant than yourselves. (Philippians 2:3)

A lover of self, however, is one with selfish love. A love of self that seeks the approval of man above all else. It looks after its own ego and pride and does not humble itself before God. Such a person does not love his eternal soul, rather he loves his sinful flesh. He does not desire the will of God, but his own will to be done. His ambitions are selfish. His motives seek to please and glorify himself.

God Leads by Example

The Lord tells us to love others as we love ourselves. He leads by example. He loves us as himself laying down his own life for ours. He respects us through his compassion and mercy, and He expects us to return that respect to him through our obedience. He respects us in our weakness and expects us to respect his authority.

Valuable or Worthy

I once heard an illustration about a $1 bill. You can crumple up, stomp on, spit on, and totally mistreat a $1 bill, but when you pick it back up, it still retains the value of one dollar. The thought was that no matter what life does to you, it doesn't take away your value. The question I debated was, "Is this true?" Can the enemy actually shred the $1 bill, (you) to a point where it is beyond repair? Can he shred your heart to a point that you lose your value.

Value is potential worth. *If you think about selling a car you may check its book value. Exchanging the car has the potential to redeem a certain amount of treasure. But it's true worth is only what the purchaser is willing to pay for it.*

*Your car may have a book **value** of $1000 but if you can only find someone willing to give you $300 for it, it is really only **worth** $300 to you, right. On the other hand, if you **believe** the car has a **value** of $4000, but if the **actual sale price** at auction is $10,000, you **underestimated its worth.** You were unable to see the value in what you had.*

*Are you valuable? Yes, you are! Every person from birth is valuable. God made each person unique and there will never be another like them in personality and character. No one else will think just like them or have the same ideas, visions, or heart. You have value because there will never be another like you with your unique traits, calling, and potential. God created you for a specific purpose which gives your life value. **Yet, the fact a person exists does not give them worth.***

What determines your worth?

The worth of something is determined by the one who redeems its value. *The one who redeemed the car for $10,000 instead of $4000, gave the car its worth. Likewise, **it is who redeems a person who gives them worth**.*

If a person tries to get their worth from the "world", they are trying to get their worth from the principalities who rule this fallen world. For the believer to seek their worth in the world, is to desire their enemy to value them, and that's not going to happen.

Do not be surprised, brothers and sisters, that the world hates you. (1 John 3:13)

To attempt to earn your value in the world, means you must seek its approval. To become friends with the world makes you God's enemy.

You adulterous people! Do you not know that friendship with the world is enmity with God? Therefore whoever wishes to be a friend of the world makes himself an enemy of God. (James 4:4)

There is no worth in our sin nature except what we give to ourselves. You will hear the world speak about "self-esteem". Why do you need to esteem yourself? Because no one in this world will esteem you, for you.

270

Worldly people will praise good deeds. So, your worth becomes entangled in your ability to be good. What happens when you screw up? They praise helpfulness and philanthropy. Your worth depends upon your ability to help others. What happens when you are the one in need? They admire success, power, and money. What happens when you fail, have financial setbacks, or someone more powerful comes along? Where does your worth go? **Your worth is at the mercy of another person's opinion.**

What happens in a world of people striving to find belonging, acceptance, and worth – anything to prove they are somehow important? You find a world full of hate. People shouting, rioting, looting, gossiping, backbiting, lying, scheming and belittling others. People who need to be seen, to matter, and have their voices heard at any cost.

Seeking value in the world places a higher and higher expectation on you to always do something more, have something more, be something better – and a person will never reach the end. They will never be enough for the world. The world will **never** *value them as they are, and their worthless pursuits will make them worthless.*

> **Thus says the LORD: "What wrong did your fathers find in me that they went far from me, and went after worthlessness, and became worthless? (Jeremiah 2:5)**

> **Now the sons of Eli were worthless men. They did not know the LORD. (1 Samuel 2:12)**

> **A worthless witness mocks at justice, and the mouth of the wicked devours iniquity. (Proverbs 19:28)**

> **Whoever loves father or mother more than me is not worthy of me, and whoever loves son or daughter more than me is not worthy of me. And whoever does not take his cross and follow me is not worthy of me. (Matthew 10:37-38)**

God's word says you have worth if *you follow Jesus, know the Lord, put nothing before Him, and follow His ways. He says you are worthless if you mock his justice, seek after worthless things or if you do not know Him.*

So, the answer to the $1 bill riddle is this.

The government is the only one with the authority to shred currency, and they only do this when taking it out of circulation. *At that point it has no worth. It can no longer be redeemed and loses all value. But* **it is illegal for anyone else to destroy** *or mutilate currency in a way that makes it worthless. The dollar bill has and retains the value it was created with as long as it is in existence.*

God is your government. *He created you and gave you your initial value, equal to every other human being. He is the authority of* **every person** *regardless of their choice to see it or not.* **He is the only One with the authority to redeem you or decommission you.** *Your worth is determined when God decides if you are righteous in Christ, or worthless chaff to be burned up in the fire. The enemy cannot redeem you. He does not have the authority to give you worth or take it away.*

The ONLY one who can determine your worth is the one who determines your fate.

The God Worthy to Give Worth

Maybe you are like me. I used to think, "It isn't that I don't trust God, I don't trust myself", or "I know that God can do anything, I'm just not sure He can with me.", or "I know God saved me, but I am too messed up to be used by Him."

While this sounds humble and faithful on the surface, in God's eyes, it shows a lack of faith. And the day I realized this; it broke my heart. You see, if God is sovereign over my life, if He changes my heart, if He makes me able, if He equips me to serve Him, if He gives and prepares me for my purpose and calling, then it is not about me at all.

What I am saying, by these seemingly humble remarks, is that I don't trust God is good enough, powerful enough, sovereign enough, to break my will. God is not stronger than I am. God can't handle me; I am too much of a challenge for Him. I was saying that God is not worthy to judge me as righteous. That is a very twisted pride.

On the other hand, I could find worth in myself from people's praise of my abilities or accomplishments. I found my worth in the people I respect standing in front of me. I saw them worthy to give me worth. Why couldn't I see God this way?

I have come in my Father's name, and you do not receive me. If another comes in his own name, you will receive him. How can you believe, when you receive glory from one another and do not seek the glory that comes from the only God? (John 5:43-44)

Let's assume that a person of importance, say a president or ruler, one that you had respect and admiration for, approached you and wanted your advice or counsel about an issue. He felt you had something to offer. He asks you to serve with him. You feel value and worth because he sees your value. You receive worth from him because you believe that he is someone worthy to give you worth.

If a street criminal asked for your advice, it is unlikely you would feel the same sense of worth. Why not? You may fear him, but you would not find him worthy of honor or respect or admiration. He is not worthy to give you worth.

Remember, God created us, and He gives us value from birth. We become worthy when we choose God. He is the one who determines if we are redeemed. When we choose His ways by faith, He takes our sin and calls us righteous. Our guilt is paid, and we do not carry shame. He redeemed us for the highest price, the cost of His own son's life. He makes us worthy. Therefore, it is the Lord who gives us both our value and our worth.

Our ability to know our worth in God is directly related to how worthy we feel God is to give us that worth and value.

How can you accept worth from someone who, in your eyes, is not worthy to give such a judgment? **if you do not find God worthy, then getting your value from him will make you feel worthless and** you would still feel the need to be validated **by someone else.**

Who do you need to validate you?

Can you see the God of the Bible as who He truly is? He is the God of complete righteousness, who orchestrates the most finite details of history. He is the God who uses each facet of creation, each person, and every situation as an instrument in His orchestra to create a symphonic masterpiece.

If the intricacies of creation and the created do not persuade you of the majesty and wisdom of our God, or the provision and acts of God in your own life do not persuade you, then certainly the unfolding of the mysteries in the Bible should leave you in utter awe!

The meaning behind every name in Biblical history, in the genealogy of Jesus, creates the story of the coming Messiah. A genealogy guarded with the lives and nation of Israel, so they could identify their Messiah, and yet just as the scriptures said, they didn't know Him. They were blind. Books written over centuries, by different authors, in a history more carefully preserved than any other history, tell a consistent story. Prophecy unfolded so perfectly and precisely hundreds and thousands of years after it was given. How does this happen without a divine all-knowing hand behind it? It cannot.

No counterfeit can do these things! See the God worthy to give you worth!

Those who lack a personal relationship with God, who do not have the Fear of the Lord and sit in awe of the majesty of who He is and what He can do, will not recognize the simple fact that He is the one who decides their fate. As such, he is the only one able to give them value, worth, and purpose. They will spend their lives seeking, and never find, and in the end be left with bitter disappointment and an eternal fate separated from God. They are burned up in the fire as worthless chaff because they refused the worth they would be so freely given, had they only accepted it.

If you still think, "It is not God who isn't worthy – its me.", are you really saying He is not worthy to make that judgment? Or are you afraid of the judgment he will make?

Remember

- *God determines if you are worthy or worthless.*
  "For behold, the day is coming, burning like a furnace; and all the arrogant and every evildoer will be chaff; and the day that is coming will set them ablaze," says the Lord of hosts, "so that it will leave them neither root nor branch."(Malachi 4:1)

- *The deciding factor is determined only by your love for God and obedience to Him.*
  And now, Israel, what does the Lord your God require of you, but to fear the Lord your God, to walk in all his ways, to love him, to serve the Lord your God with all your heart and with all your soul, (Deuteronomy 10:12)

Man-made Truth

Defining religion is controversial and therefore difficult. Perhaps it can be best defined as a person's beliefs, values, and practices based on the teachings of a spiritual leader. The world is always creating its own religions or "world-views". Even if the belief is atheism (that there is no God or higher power) you have a religion. Think about it. If your beliefs, values, and practices are based on the teaching that there is an absence of a spiritual being, this is still a spiritual belief. Not only does the world deny God, but it also redefines Him and His ways as it sees fit.

As a Christian, you are probably very aware that worship of false gods, witchcraft, and idolatry are sins that have a steep and eternal consequence from the Lord. There are many specific things described in scripture that fall into these categories The obvious ones include sacrificing your child in the fire, divination or sorcery, witchcraft, spells, consulting or being a medium or spiritualist, consulting the dead, or interpreting omens. These people create their own truth apart from the Lord. Anyone who does these things is detestable to Him. You may think all Christians are far removed from witchcraft and idolatry as described in the scriptures, but let's take a deeper look.

Occultic Christians?

Christians are no less guilty of defining truth than the world. Some ways are easy to spot through scripture. Perhaps you know of Christians who talk about deceased loved ones as their guardian angels, or who worship angels. God created the angels. They serve Him and minister to us. They watch us with interest because we are created in the image of their creator! We are not, nor do we become angels. Angel worship is idol worship.

> **And to which of the angels has he ever said, "Sit at my right hand until I make your enemies a footstool for your feet"? Are they not all ministering spirits sent out to serve for the sake of those who are to inherit salvation? (Hebrews1:13-14)**

> **It was revealed to them that they were serving not themselves but you, in the things that have now been announced to you through those who preached the good news to you by the Holy Spirit sent from heaven, things into which angels long to look.**
> **(1 Peter 1:12)**

Perhaps you have heard a Christian talk about seeing or speaking to the spirit of a dead relative. Desperate for answers and healing, some believe this is a gifting from God, but the Bible clearly teaches that the dead and living cannot communicate. This is like consulting a medium. These people are deceived and communicating with demons.

> **"And he said, 'No, father Abraham, but if someone goes to them from the dead, they will repent.' He said to him, 'If they do not hear Moses and the Prophets, neither will they be convinced if someone should rise from the dead.'" (Luke 16:30-31)**

Unfortunately, Satan has also infiltrated God's church in more subtle ways. He may not fool you with a blatant deception. He often deceives with partial truth.

I often hear Christians talk about karma? Some churches even offer Yoga for health, discounting it as a spiritual ritual. Yoga was first used by Brahmans, Vedic priests, and Rishis, who are mystic seers. It internalized the idea of ritual sacrifice, teaching the sacrifice of the ego through self-knowledge and action (karma yoga) and wisdom (jnana yoga). Karma is the antithesis of God's grace and the foundations of a false religion.

Many Christians discount pagan and occultic things as just fun. They see no harm in playing with a Ouija board, discounting that they open a real gateway to communicate with the demonic. "It is just a game sold in kid's stores."

They may play video or role-playing games that have spiritualism built in. They may read books or watch videos, television, or movies with vampires, demons, occult activity, or lude behavior. They may listen to music with lyrics that counter God's word, believing it is okay because they "know the truth" and they don't believe in these things.

Have you ever had your palm read at a festival? Do you pay attention to your astrological sign or look at your horoscope? Do you interpret omens, or interpret a circumstance to influence your actions? Do you rely on lucky numbers or keep good luck charms? These are occultic activities that replace prayer and discernment from God.

Is This Simply Overreacting to Harmless Fun?

Satan uses the media to manipulate. There is little you can watch or listen to in entertainment that is not immersed with what God finds abhorrent. **Perhaps you don't see the problem with watching a television show** that has some lude behavior, vampires, demons, or occult activity. Maybe they are cute-ified, like a kids show with a puppy that finds a spell book and innocently reads an incantation, **but it has a moral story!** So, you allow your children to watch it.

What would the God, that you read about in scripture, think about Christian children being entertained by the occult simply because they are not practicing it? Does that even make sense to you? This is like saying that it is okay to watch pornography because you are not physically engaged in it. **Not being physically engaged** in an act of immorality **does not mean that your heart is not engaged in it.**

> **And he said, "What comes out of a person is what defiles him. For from within, out of the heart of man, come evil thoughts, sexual immorality, theft, murder, adultery, coveting, wickedness, deceit, sensuality, envy, slander, pride, foolishness. All these evil things come from within, and they defile a person." (Mark 7:20-23)**

Satan is the prince of the air. He uses what we see and hear to sugar coat and delude the masses. He comes to devour like a roaring lion. **He wants that show to corrupt your child.** He wants that inuendo in that song to stick in your child's brain so when he reaches maturity it can have its full effect.

What we take into our minds becomes part of us, and the Lord warns us to only set our minds on what is right.

Finally, brothers, whatever is true, whatever is honorable, whatever is just, whatever is pure, whatever is lovely, whatever is commendable, if there is any excellence, if there is anything worthy of praise, think about these things. What you have learned and received and heard and seen in me—practice these things, and the God of peace will be with you. (Philippians 4:8-9)

Do not allow your mind to be filled with distractions of everything in the world around you through news or social media. God wants us to look at Him, not all the deception circling around us like vultures. Amazingly, you will not be uninformed about what you need to know. Remember He is sovereign, not us, so knowing all the spin changes nothing.

Redefining God's Truth in the Church

There is much falsehood in the church today. It was a slow progression. Now it is hard to know what truth is. Who is the real God? Without the Holy Spirit helping you discern the scripture; you will be deceived. Test everything you read or hear in a sermon or music against the truth of God's word.

And they shall turn away their ears from the truth and shall be turned unto fables (2 Timothy 4:4).

In the 1950's, Science tried to replace God. Apologetics came about and tried to fight it, but by the 1960's the church faced moral issues and did not stand. They chose to be tolerant, but tolerating sin is not loving the sinner. They let sin go, and what started as ignoring sin, evolved in the church. Now many denominations of the church embrace sin as righteousness and God turns them over.

Both things continue as we walk forward in the original sin, defining for ourselves what is right and wrong and determining for ourselves what is truth. There is only one who defines truth. Only one who defines good and evil. And that is the LORD.

Today, the church has people embracing false, demonic, spirits masquerading as the Holy Spirit of God. People performing false miracles for a price, getting rich off the backs of desperate believers. Political social justice warriors have hitched a ride on the back of faith in an attempt to hijack a movement and gain power. Some churches embrace a greezy-feel-good-grace doctrine, refusing to preach any message that may offend, shouting legalism at the mention of morality, and leading people straight to hell.

A prosperity doctrine has infiltrated the church that drives people into depression or away from God because their success with Christ is dependent upon their ability to believe enough. The theology is one that implies you don't have what you want, not because of sin or because God has different plans, but because you are not believing enough. This leaves a person believing they are not good enough and a failure with God.

Legalistic doctrine completely dismisses the Spirit of God, dismisses women, dismisses the prophetic, or that any new thing could happen because it has already been done. They believe the word is all we have; God no longer speaks to his people. That is not truth!

A false, misleading, representation of our God and His word has people chasing signs and a goose-bump feeling. The Lord does confirm his thoughts and ways to us, but when the Lord gives you a sign, you should be able to back up what he is saying and how he is saying it, in the scripture. He will show you. God doesn't change, and the way He speaks to His people does not change either, yet our ability to hear him certainly has changed.

It is more important than ever to be solid in your word.

- *Do not lean on prior understanding or teachings. Let the Lord teach you.*

- *Do not allow yourself to be spoon-fed the scripture from pastors or books.*

- *Seek the Holy Spirit as you read the Word of God for yourself!*

- *Learn the word. Read it all, and then read it again to study it deeper.*

- *Seek differences in translations and research the original language used.*

- *Learn about types and shadows in scripture.*

- *Allow the Holy Spirit to give understanding of parables.*

- *Take every verse in context with the entirety of scripture.*

- *Understand the original Jewish perspective of the passage you are reading.*

- *Use surveys of the Old and New Testament to learn about the culture and history of the time in which the scripture was written.*

Regret

What more can a man do about yesterday,
than what He does, when the Lord makes everything new.

Then I saw a new heaven and a new earth, for the first heaven and the first earth had passed away, and the sea was no more. And I saw the holy city, new Jerusalem, coming down out of heaven from God, prepared as a bride adorned for her husband. And I heard a loud voice from the throne saying, "Behold, the dwelling place of God is with man. He will dwell with them, and they will be his people, and God himself will be with them as their God. He will wipe away every tear from their eyes, and death shall be no more, neither shall there be mourning, nor crying, nor pain anymore, for the former things have passed away." And he who was seated on the throne said, "Behold, I am making all things new." Also he said, "Write this down, for these words are trustworthy and true." And he said to me, "It is done! I am the Alpha and the Omega, the beginning and the end. To the thirsty I will give from the spring of the water of life without payment. The one who conquers will have this heritage, and I will be his God and he will be my son. (Revelation 21:1-7)

"Behold, I am coming soon, bringing my recompense with me, to repay each one for what he has done. I am the Alpha and the Omega, the first and the last, the beginning and the end." Blessed are those who wash their robes, so that they may have the right to the tree of life and that they may enter the city by the gates. Outside are the dogs and sorcerers and the sexually immoral and murderers and idolaters, and everyone who loves and practices falsehood. "I, Jesus, have sent my angel to testify to you about these things for the churches. I am the root and the descendant of David, the bright morning star." The Spirit and the Bride say, "Come." And let the one who hears say, "Come." And let the one who is thirsty come; let the one who desires take the water of life without price. (Revelation 22:12-17)

And this is the will of him who sent me, that I should lose nothing of all that he has given me, but raise it up on the last day. For this is the will of my Father, that everyone who looks on the Son and believes in him should have eternal life, and I will raise him up on the last day." (John 6:39-40)

Visit the website at:

www.rebuiltrecovery.org

for downloadable pages and
more helpful resources!